Clinical Ultrasound

Case Reviews

Edward Hoey, MB BCh BAO MRCP FRCR
Cardiothoracic Imaging Fellow
Papworth Hospital, Cambridge, UK

Jane Alty, MB BChir MA MRCP
Specialist Registrar
Leeds General Infirmary Hospital, Leeds, UK

Kshitij Mankad, MB BCh MRCP MBA
Specialist Registrar
Leeds and West Yorkshire Radiology Academy
Leeds, UK

Guest Editors

Andrew Scarsbrook, BMedSci BM BS FRCR
Consultant Radiologist

Rosemary Arthur, MBChB Bsc MRCP FRCR
Consultant Paediatric Radiologist

Leeds Teaching Hospitals NHS Trust, Leeds, UK

CLINICAL ULTRASOUND
Case Reviews

Published in the UK by:

Anshan Ltd
11a Little Mount Sion
Tunbridge Wells
Kent. TN1 1YS

Tel: +44 (0) 1892 557767
Fax: +44 (0) 1892 530358

e-mail: info@anshan.co.uk
web site: www.anshan.co.uk

© 2011 Edward Hoey, Jane Alty

ISBN: 978 1 848290 49 5

The use of registered names, trademarks, etc, in this publication does not imply, even in the absence of a specific statement that such names are exempt from the relevant laws and regulations and therefore for general use.

While every effort has been made to ensure the accuracy of the information contained within this publication, the publisher can give no guarantee for information about drug dosage and application thereof contained in this book. In every individual case the respective user must check current indications and accuracy by consulting other pharmaceutical literature and following the guidelines laid down by the manufacturers of specific products and the relevant authorities in the country in which they are practicing.

British Library Cataloguing in Publication Data
A catalogue record for this book is available from the British Library.

Copy Editor: Andrew White
Cover Design: Emma Randall
Cover Image: Edward Hoey
Typeset by: GCS, Leighton Buzzard, Bedfordshire, LU7 1EU

Contents

Preface

Ultrasound is a demanding specialty requiring an in-depth knowledge of anatomy, physics and pathology as well as many hours of practical scanning experience. Trainees are required to attain high levels of competency in a relatively short period of time and ultrasound images play an ever increasing role in the radiology fellowship examinations.

This book has been written to give trainees exposure to a wide range of ultrasound pathologies and has been compiled in a question-and-answer format to aid with exam preparation. In most instances there is a specific answer, but in some a limited differential diagnosis is required. Selected images with typical accompanying case histories are provided and are followed by a labelled image and summary of the salient diagnostic features of that condition. Some 'hints' are included to aid with day-to-day practice.

Although specifically aimed at radiology trainees, this series of case reviews will also be useful to sonographers, physicians, medical students and anyone with an interest in ultrasound.

Edward Hoey
Jane Alty
Kshitij Mankad

Acknowledgements

We would like to thank our friends and families for their help and support during the writing and editing of this book. We also thank all the consultants and sonographers based at the Leeds Teaching Hospitals for their guidance and training during our placements.

Thanks also to Teresa Humphrey for editing paediatric case 8.

Chapter 1

Renal and Renal Transplant

CASE 1

A patient is referred 3 days post–renal transplant with oliguria.

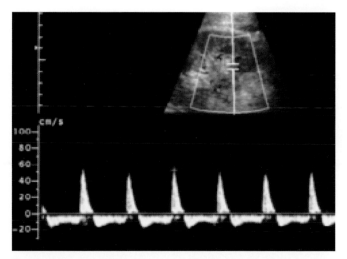

Transplant inter-lobar artery (ILA) spectral Doppler

Q1. What is the diagnosis?

A1. Renal vein thrombosis

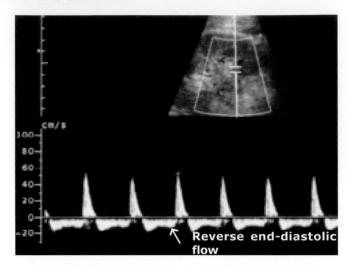

Notes

Renal vein thrombosis is an uncommon, but serious early transplant complication.

Predisposing factors include faulty surgical anastomosis and transplant compression by peri-renal fluid collections. Patients will be oliguric with a tender, swollen graft.

Ultrasound Features
• Swollen kidney with subcapsular fluid collections.
• Absent colour flow in the main renal vein.
• Inter-lobar artery Doppler waveform shows reverse end-diastolic flow.

Hints

Renal vein thrombosis renders the transplant non-viable and is a surgical emergency.

CASE 2

A 19-year-old man presents with haematuria, proteinuria and renal failure.

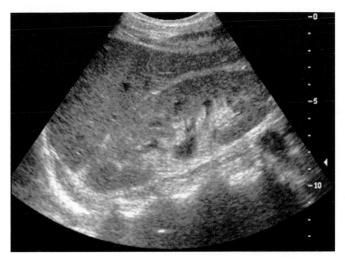

LS right kidney/liver

Q1. What is the diagnosis?

A1. Acute renal parenchymal disease

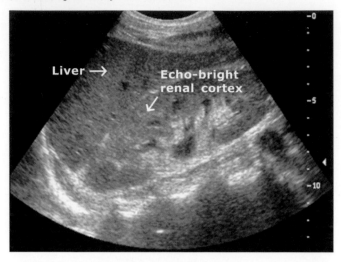

Notes

There are many causes of renal parenchymal disease including acute tubular necrosis (e.g., iodinated contrast reaction) and acute glomerulonephritis.

Ultrasound Features

- Swollen echo-bright renal cortex.
- Prominent medullary pyramids (punched-out pyramids sign).
- Raised inter-lobar artery resistance index (>0.7).
- The kidneys may have a normal appearance.

Hints

Look for intra-peritoneal free fluid (secondary to low protein state) in Morrison's pouch, both flanks, and in the pelvis.

Ultrasound cannot specify the aetiology, and clinical correlation is essential.

Ultrasound-guided renal biopsy may be used to provide a histological diagnosis.

CASE 3

A 60-year-old man under investigation for haematuria is referred for renal ultrasound.

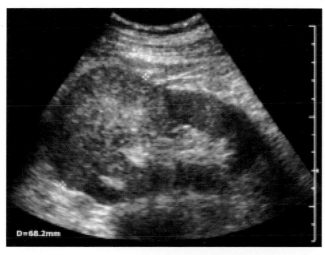

LS left kidney

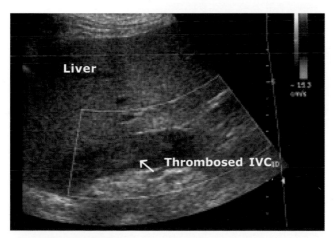

LS inferior vena cava (colour Doppler)

Q1. What is the diagnosis?
Q2. What complication has occurred?

A1. Renal cell carcinoma
A2. Inferior vena cava invasion

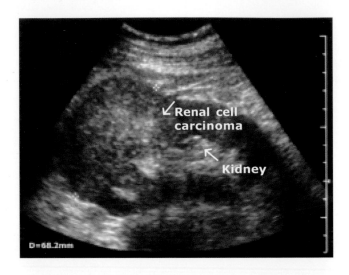

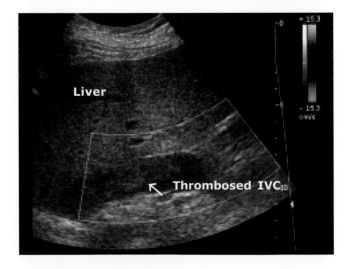

Notes
Renal cell carcinoma (RCC) is the commonest renal malignancy in adults. Predisposing factors include long-term dialysis, tuberous sclerosis and von Hippel-Lindau disease. It classically presents with

a clinical triad of haematuria, loin pain and an abdominal mass. RCC has a propensity for invasion into the renal vein and vena cava (IVC) which must be carefully interrogated using colour Doppler.

Ultrasound Features
- Mixed echogenicity mass lesion causing a renal contour bulge.
- Small tumours appear echo-bright and can mimic angiomyolipomas.
- Renal vein and IVC invasion appears as an expanded thrombus-filled vein with absent colour flow on Doppler interrogation.

Hints
Renal vein invasion is seen as an expanded vein containing echo-bright thrombus.

Rarely a left-sided RCC can obstruct the left testicular vein causing a varicocele.

The other kidney should be inspected carefully as 5% are bilateral.

CASE 4

A 50-year-old man with hypertension refractory to drug treatment is referred for renal ultrasound.

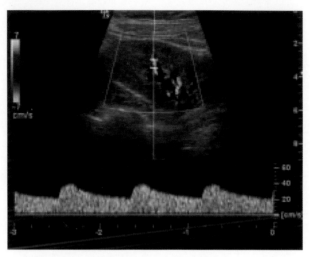

Right kidney ILA spectral Doppler

Q1. What does this Doppler waveform demonstrate?
Q2. What is the diagnosis?

A1. Parvus tardus waveform
A2. Renal artery stenosis

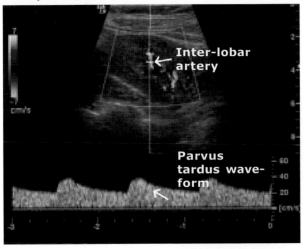

Notes

Renal artery stenosis (RAS) causes a reduced perfusion pressure at the glomerulus which stimulates renin production leading to a rise in angiotensin which in turn causes a rise in blood pressure. It accounts for 2–5% of all cases of hypertension. Clinically it presents with hypertension refractory to drug treatment, renal failure or both. RAS is considered haemodynamically significant when there is >70% narrowing of the lumen. Most stenoses are caused by atherosclerosis, but fibromuscular dysplasia and neurofibromatosis are other recognised associations. Diagnosis can be made via angiography or from Doppler ultrasound interrogation of the renal arteries. Balloon angioplasty is an established treatment option.

Ultrasound Features

- Unilateral small kidney
- Main renal artery peak systolic velocity >180 cm/s
- Ratio of peak systolic renal velocity to aortic velocity >3.5
- 'Parvus tardus' inter-lobar artery Doppler waveform

Hints

An inter-lobar artery Doppler waveform acceleration time >0.07 is considered diagnostic of significant RAS. Although Doppler ultrasound has a high sensitivity for RAS its specificity is low and it cannot 'rule out' the diagnosis. Further imaging with magnetic resonance or catheter angiography is required in these cases.

CASE 5

A 45-year-old woman with a hereditary kidney disorder presents with left-sided abdominal pain.

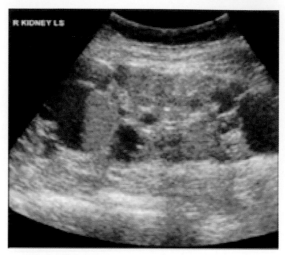

LS left kidney

Q1. What is the diagnosis?
Q2. What complication has occurred?

A1. Adult polycystic kidney disease
A2. Cyst haemorrhage

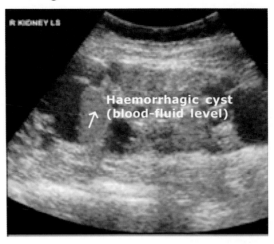

Notes
Adult polycystic kidney disease (APKD) is relatively common and transmitted as an autosomal dominant trait. Microscopic cysts are present in the nephrons at birth and slowly accumulate fluid increasing in size with age. Presentation is usually in the 4th or 5th decade with bilateral flank masses, hypertension and progressive renal failure. Common complications include cyst haemorrhage, infection or rupture into the perinephric space.

Ultrasound Features
• Enlarged kidneys with an undulating surface.
• Contain multiple cysts of varying sizes.
• Haemorrhage or infection cause more complex-looking cysts.

Hints
Hepatic cystic disease is a common concomitant finding. Pancreatic and splenic cysts are less common.

Cerebral aneurysms are present in 10–15% of patients and subarachnoid haemorrhage is occasionally the initial mode of presentation.

CASE 6

A 45-year-old man is having a renal ultrasound for investigation of haematuria.

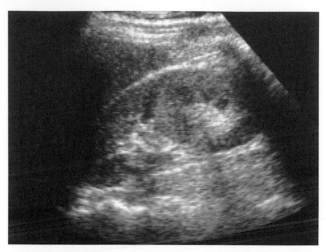

LS left kidney

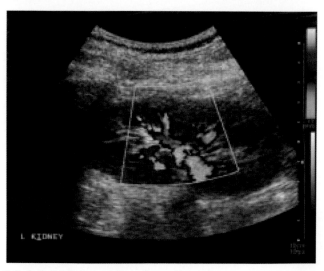

LS left kidney with colour Doppler

Q1. What is the diagnosis?
Q2. What condition can mimic it?

A1. Column of Bertin
A2. Renal cell carcinoma

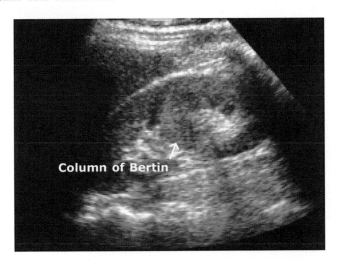

Notes
Column of Bertin is hypertrophy of a column of cortex which protrudes into the renal sinus fat. It is a normal variation in renal morphology and should not be confused with a renal cell carcinoma.

Ultrasound Features
Distinguishing features versus renal cell carcinoma
- Mass is in continuity with the cortex.
- Mass is of the same echogenicity as the cortex.
- Mass does not cause any distortion of the renal contour.

Hints
Colour Doppler assessment shows the lesion has normal vascularity unlike renal cell carcinoma which is hypervascular.

CASE 7

A 40-year-old man who had a kidney transplant 2 months ago is referred for ultrasound because of low urine output and rising urea and creatinine levels.

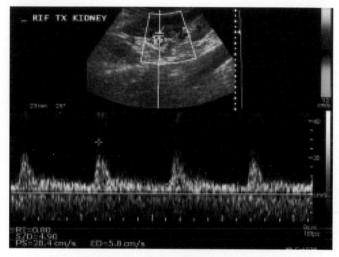

Transplant ILA spectral Doppler

Q1. What does this Doppler waveform demonstrate?
Q2. What is the differential diagnosis?

A1. Low diastolic flow with raised resistance index
A2. Acute rejection or cyclosporine drug toxicity

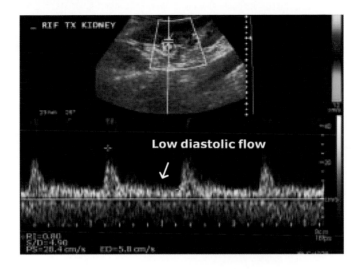

Notes
Acute Rejection
This is mediated via cellular immunity with lymphocytic and polymorphonuclear infiltrates. It most commonly occurs during the first 6 months following transplantation. Most cases can be successfully treated using pulsed corticosteroids.

Cyclosporine Toxicity
This is mediated via a direct nephrotoxic effect and most commonly occurs during the first 2–3 months when drug levels are highest.

Ultrasound Features
There are no specific features to distinguish between the two conditions.
- Swollen kidney
- Echo-bright renal cortex
- Reduced brightness of renal sinus fat
- Elevated resistance index (>0.7)

Hints
Always ensure the bladder is empty prior to measuring the resistance index as back pressure effects make it artificially high.

Ultrasound-guided renal biopsy is used to distinguish rejection from drug toxicity.

Serial resistance index measurements are more helpful than a single value when monitoring transplants.

CASE 8

A 50-year-old man who had a renal transplant 1 year ago is referred for ultrasound because of rising urea and creatinine levels. The transplant ureter was stented 6 months previously because of an anastomotic stricture.

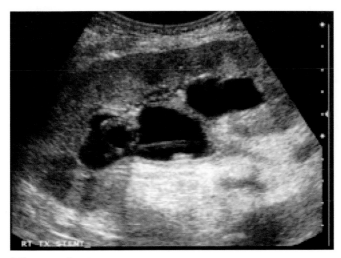

LS transplant

Q1. What is the diagnosis?
Q2. What treatment is needed?

A1. Ureteric stent blockage
A2. The stent needs to be replaced

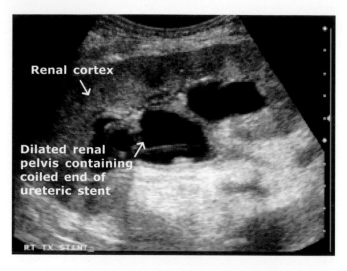

Notes

Ureteric stents are commonly used to treat anastomotic strictures which occur at the bladder wall. The stent may subsequently block with debris or blood clot leading to graft dysfunction. Urgent replacement is needed to prevent irreversible graft damage.

Ultrasound Features

- Transplant pelvicalyceal system dilatation.
- Resistance index will be raised from back pressure effects.
- Absent ureteric jet using colour Doppler.

Hints

Always ensure the bladder is empty before assessment of the collecting system as back pressure effects can mimic obstruction.

A mild degree of pelvicalyceal system dilatation in the first postoperative week is considered normal and is caused by oedema at the anastomotic site.

CASE 9

A 35-year-old man is having a routine abdominal ultrasound.

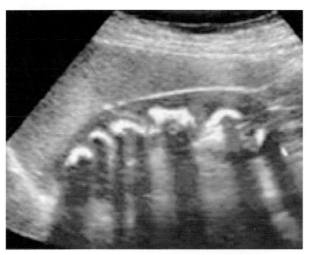

LS right kidney

Q1. What is the diagnosis?
Q2. What is the likely cause?

A1. Medullary nephrocalcinosis
A2. Medullary sponge kidney

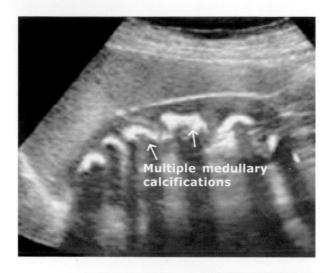

Notes

Nephrocalcinosis is the deposition of calcium salts within the renal parenchyma. Most cases occur in the medulla where causes include hyperparathyroidism, medullary sponge kidney and type 1 renal tubular acidosis. Medullary sponge kidney is the development of ectatic tubules in the medullary pyramids leading to urinary stasis and stone formation. Most patients are asymptomatic and have normal renal function.

Ultrasound Features

- Multiple echo-bright areas within the medullary pyramids
- Display post-acoustic shadowing

Hints

Cortical nephrocalcinosis is rare. Causes include sickle cell disease, acute cortical necrosis, chronic glomerulonephritis and oxalosis.

CASE 10

A 58-year-old woman with fevers, chills and right-sided loin pain is referred for ultrasound.

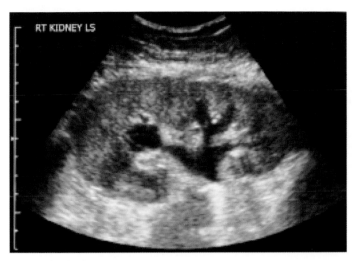

LS right kidney

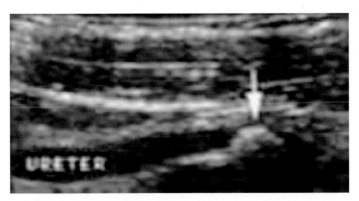

LS distal right ureter

Q1. What is the diagnosis?
Q2. What complication has occurred?

A1. Obstructive uropathy (stone at VUJ)
A2. Pyonephrosis

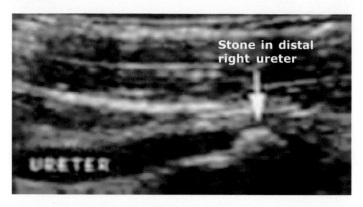

Notes

Pyonephrosis is infected purulent urine in an obstructed collecting system. Obstruction is most often caused by a calculus or tumour and *E.coli* is the commonest cultured organism. Patients are systemically unwell with fever and rigors. Pyonephrosis requires urgent drainage to prevent overwhelming sepsis and cardiovascular collapse.

Ultrasound Features
• Hydronephrosis
• Echogenic debris with the collecting system
• Reverberation artefacts seen with gas-forming organisms

Hints

Percutaneous nephrostomy tube placement allows drainage of an infected system and treatment planning once the patient is stable.

CASE 11

A 45-year-old woman is being investigated for haematuria and right-sided loin pain.

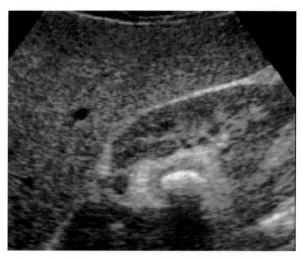

LS right kidney

Q1. What is the diagnosis?

A1. Renal stone

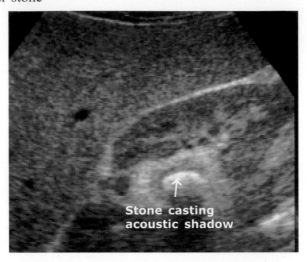

Stone casting acoustic shadow

Notes

Most urinary stones are composed of calcium mixed with oxalate, phosphate or a combination of the two. Struvite stones (magnesium ammonium phosphate) make up around 15% and form in the presence of infection. Cystine, urate and xanthine stones are rare. Stones are prone to pass into and obstruct the ureter. Those >6 mm are unlikely to pass spontaneously and usually require some form of interventional removal.

Ultrasound Features
- Echo-bright focus that casts a distal acoustic shadow
- Hydronephrosis if lodged in the ureter

Hints

Increasing the frequency and reducing the overall gain makes stone detection easier.

Stones may be difficult to detect if obscured by renal sinus echoes; always look for post-acoustic shadowing as a clue.

Always measure the size of any stones and note their location.

CASE 12

A 60-year-old man is having a renal ultrasound for investigation of possible renal stones.

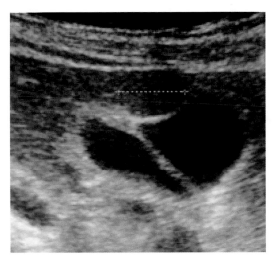

LS left renal cortex

Q1. What is the diagnosis?

A1. Complex renal cyst

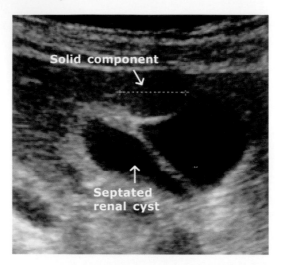

Notes

Renal cysts are commonly encountered lesions. Benign 'simple' cysts may be complicated by haemorrhage or infection giving them a more complex appearance and any cyst with atypical features must be differentiated from a renal cell carcinoma. The presence of multiple internal septations, thick septations or wall nodularity all warrant excision for histological assessment as per the Bosniak classification system.

Ultrasound Features
Simple benign cyst (Ignore)
- Thin walled
- Smooth edge
- Echo-free contents
- Fine (<1 mm) internal septations
- Small punctuate calcifications

Atypical features (Requires follow-up or excision)
- Thick internal septations
- Solid components
- Thick nodular calcifications

Hints

CT or MRI assessment should be used in conjunction with ultrasound in the assessment of a suspicious cystic renal lesion. Septal or wall enhancement following intravenous contrast administration indicates an aggressive lesion requiring surgical excision.

CASE 13

A 55-year-old diabetic woman presents with right flank pain, fevers and is septic with *E.coli* grown in her blood cultures.

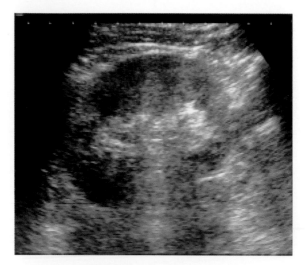

LS right kidney

Q1. What is causing the shadowing?
Q2. What is the diagnosis?

A1. Gas in the renal parenchyma
A2. Emphysematous pyelonephritis

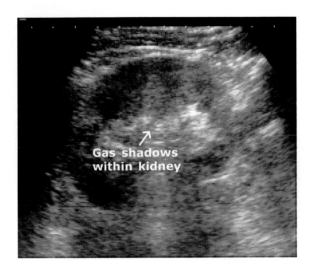

Notes
Emphysematous pyelonephritis is a fulminant necrotizing infection of the renal parenchyma caused by gas-forming organisms. It primarily affects patients with diabetes or severe immunosuppression. *E.coli* is the commonest pathogen. Patients are profoundly unwell with flank pain, positive blood cultures and sepsis. Treatment is nephrectomy and intravenous antibiotics, but the prognosis is grave with up to 80% mortality.

Ultrasound Features
- Reverberation artefacts (gas) in the parenchyma

Hints
Gas shadows are 'dirty' whereas calculi cast a 'clean' acoustic shadow. In severe cases there may be so much gas shadowing that the kidney cannot be visualised and if there is clinical suspicion the patient should have a CT scan to establish the diagnosis.

CASE 14

A 45-year-old man with end-stage renal failure on haemodialysis is being worked up for renal transplantation.

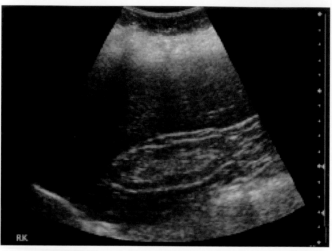

LS right kidney

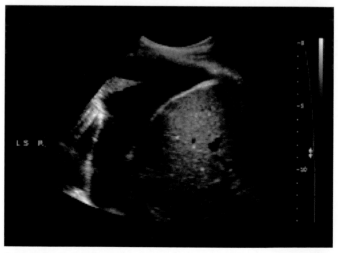

LS right lobe liver

Q1. What is the kidney appearance typical of?
Q2. What other observation is there?

A1. Chronic renal failure
A2. Right pleural effusion

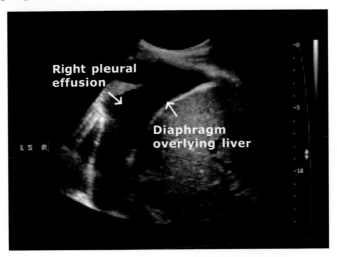

Notes
Chronic renal failure is a long standing loss of function over months to years. Causes include chronic glomerulonephritis and diabetic/ hypertensive nephropathy.

Ultrasound Features
- Kidneys are small with a thinned cortex (may be difficult to find them).
- Inter-lobar artery resistance index is elevated.

Hints
Look for other signs of renal failure such as ascites and pleural effusions.

If a kidney cannot be found, there are three possibilities:
- It is present but hidden, e.g., small atrophic kidney or abundance of bowel gas
- It is in an ectopic location
- It is absent

Chapter 2

Gallbladder, Pancreas & Spleen

CASE 1

A 17-year-old man with sickle cell anaemia is referred with intermittent RUQ pain.

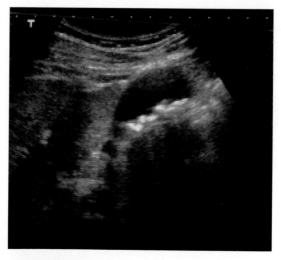

LS RUQ

Q1. What is the diagnosis?

A1. Pigment gallstones

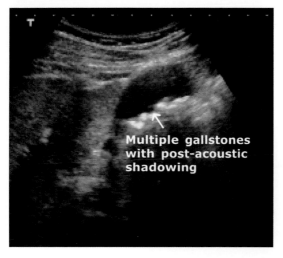

Notes

Pigment stones account for 10–20% of all gallstones. They are associated with states of excessive red blood cell destruction as occurs in haemolytic anaemias. As with other types of gallstones they may present with recurrent episodes of biliary colic or simply be chance incidental findings at ultrasonography. Pigment stones tend to be smaller and more numerous than the other stone types.

Ultrasound Features
- Echo-bright intraluminal lesions
- Cast a distal acoustic shadow
- Gravity dependant

Hints

Complications of gallstones include cholecystitis and pancreatitis.

Increasing the machine frequency setting and reducing the overall gain makes stones more conspicuous.

CASE 2

A 40-year-old woman is referred for routine abdominal ultrasound.

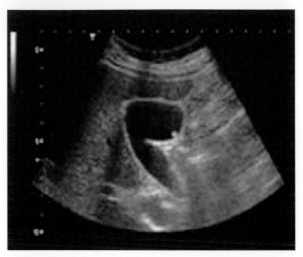

LS gallbladder

Q1. What does this image show?

A1. Gallblader polyp

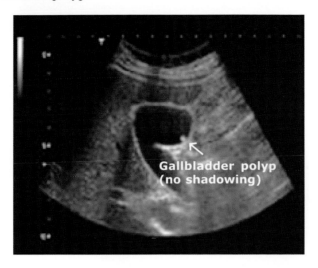

Notes

Gallbladder polyps are a common finding, occurring in around 5% of the population. They are usually asymptomatic, but large polyps can be associated with malignant transformation into gallbladder carcinoma.

Ultrasound Features
- Well-defined wall-based lesion
- No post-acoustic shadowing
- Not gravity dependant

Hints

Polyps can be distinguished from gallstones by rescanning the patient in a different position. Stones will move as they are gravity dependant but polyps remain fixed.

Solitary, large (>8 mm) polyps should be considered adenomatous (premalignant) and warrant surgical referral for cholecystectomy.

CASE 3

A 72-year-old woman with a past history of gallstones presents with a 2-month history of right upper quadrant pain.

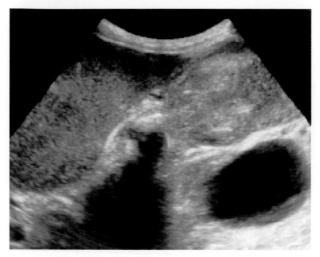

LS gallbladder

Q1. What is the diagnosis?

A1. Gallbladder carcinoma

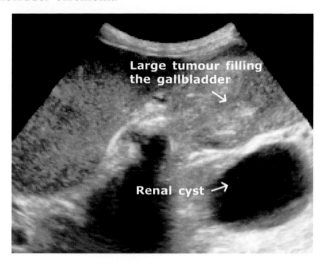

Notes
Gallbladder carcinoma is a highly malignant tumour of the gallbladder wall. It is most prevalent in elderly females and associated with chronic cholecystitis, porcelain gallbladder and large polyps (>8 mm). The majority are locally invasive and unresectable at time of diagnosis. The mean survival time is only 6 months.

Ultrasound Features
- Associated with gallstones
- Gallbladder wall thickening in early disease
- Gallbladder replaced by a mixed echogenicity mass in late disease
- Invasion into adjacent liver parenchyma

Hints
The dire prognosis from these tumours highlights the importance of early detection and cholecystectomy for large polyps.

CASE 4

A 60-year-old man presents with weight loss and painless jaundice.

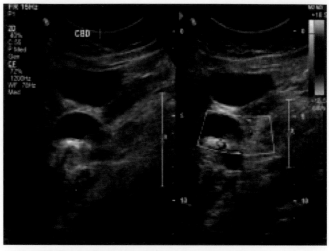

LS CBD

Q1. What is the diagnosis?

A1. Cholangiocarcinoma

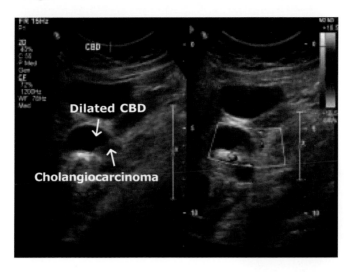

Notes

Cholangiocarcinoma is a malignant tumour arising from the epithelial lining of the bile ducts. It occurs most frequently in an extrahepatic location. Predisposing factors include clonorchis (liver fluke) infestation, choledochal cysts and sclerosing cholangitis. Cholangiocarcinoma presents with symptoms and signs of biliary tree obstruction.

Ultrasound Features (extrahepatic cholangiocarcinoma)
Early
- Irregular thickening of bile duct wall
- Proximal biliary ductal dilatation

Late
- Ill-defined tumour mass at the site of obstruction

Hints

Early extrahepatic tumours can be indistinguishable from sclerosing cholangitis which also causes irregular wall thickening of the CBD. ERCP with biopsy is required in such cases.

Tumour invasion into adjacent structures (liver, pancreas, portal vein) indicates advanced stage disease and precludes surgical resection.

CASE 5

A 55-year-old woman is referred with longstanding RUQ pain.

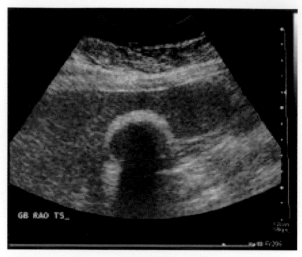

TS gallbladder

Q1. What is the diagnosis?
Q2. What disease does this predispose to?

A1. Porcelain gallbladder
A2. Gallbladder carcinoma

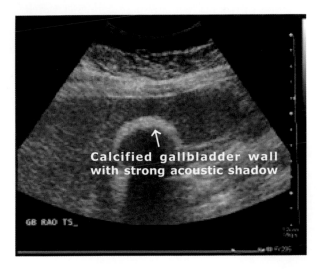

Calcified gallbladder wall with strong acoustic shadow

GB RAO TS

Notes
Porcelain gallbladder refers to dystrophic calcification of a chronically inflamed gallbladder wall and is nearly always associated with gallstones. The condition merits a cholecystectomy as up to 25% of patients subsequently develop a gallbladder carcinoma.

Ultrasound Features
• Echo-bright curvilinear structure in the gallbladder fossa
• Casts a strong acoustic shadow
• Obscures visualisation of gallbladder contents

Hints
The main differential diagnosis is of a contracted gallbladder full of stones.

In this condition look for the anterior gallbladder wall as a separate structure from the stones. This is the 'double arc shadow sign'. It may be necessary to scan the patient in a variety of positions to achieve this.

CASE 6

A 50-year-old man presents with jaundice, fevers and RUQ pains.

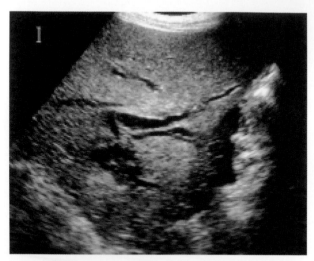

LS left lobe liver

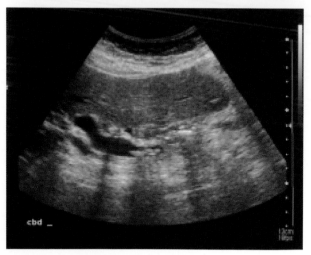

LS distal CBD

Q1. What is the diagnosis?
Q2. What has caused this?

A1. Ascending cholangitis
A2. Impacted stones in the CBD

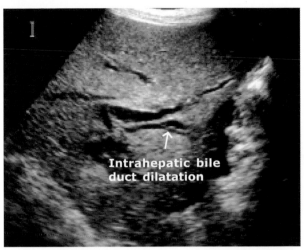

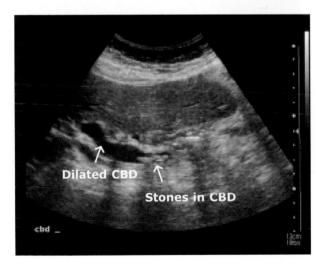

Notes
Ascending cholangitis is a bacterial infection of the biliary tree and is usually caused by a stone lodging in the distal bile duct which acts as a nidus for infection. Untreated it leads to hepatic abscesses, septicaemia and is uniformly fatal. Ultrasound is used to detect the biliary obstruction and can often pin point its cause.

Ultrasound Features

Dilated biliary tree proximal to the level of obstruction

- CBD >6 mm.
- Intrahepatic duct dilatation.
- Echo-bright stone may be seen lodged in the CBD.

Hints

Gas in the 1st and 2nd parts of the duodenum can obscure visualisation of the distal CBD where stones commonly lodge. Scanning patients in the left lateral position and using the gallbladder as a window can help visualise this area better.

MRCP or ERCP may be required to make the diagnosis.

CASE 7

A 50-year-old woman presents with RUQ pain, vomiting, fever and raised inflammatory markers.

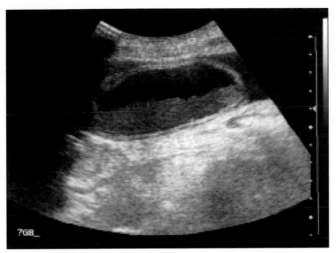

LS gallbladder

Q1. What is the diagnosis?

A1. Acute cholecystitis

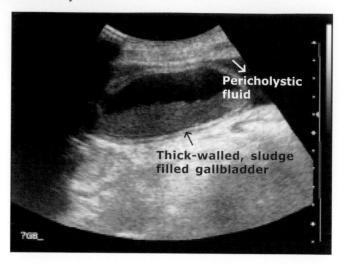

Notes
Cholecystitis is inflammation of the gallbladder wall. Most cases are caused by impacted stones/sludge in the gallbladder neck or cystic duct. Acalculous cholecystitis is sometimes seen in the critical care setting.

Ultrasound Features
- Tender distended gallbladder
- Gallstones or sludge (95% of cases)
- Gallbladder wall thickness >3 mm
- Oedematous wall with indistinct outline
- Rim of echo-free pericholecystic fluid

Hints
Gallbladder wall thickening is a fairly non-specific sign by itself as there are a wide range of causes including hepatitis, ascites, heart failure and AIDS.

Reverberation artefact (gas) in the gallbladder wall represents a particularly severe form of infection (emphysematous cholecystitis) and is associated with a high risk of perforation.

CASE 8

A 60-year-old man with anaemia is referred for an abdominal ultrasound.

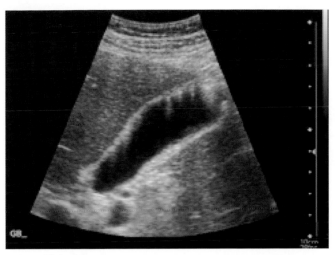

LS gallbladder

Q1. What is this incidental finding?

A1. Adenomyomatosis

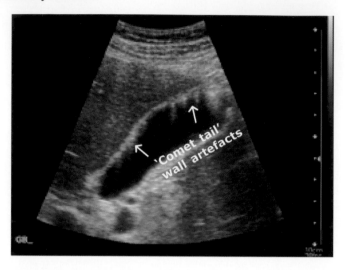

Notes
This benign condition is associated with gallstones. There is hyperplasia of the gallbladder wall epithelium resulting in mucosal diverticulae that extend into the muscular layer. The diverticulae are seen within the wall as fluid or crystal-filled spaces.

Ultrasound Features
- GB wall thickening can be diffuse or focal.
- Diverticulae containing bile are echo-poor.
- Diverticulae containing stones/sludge give a 'comet tail' artefact.

Hints
Adenomyomatosis usually causes generalised gallbladder wall thickening, but can be focal, particularly at the fundus where it is termed an adenomyoma. This can mimic the appearance of an early gallbladder carcinoma.

CASE 9

A 40-year-old woman is suffering from recurrent episodes of hypoglycaemia.

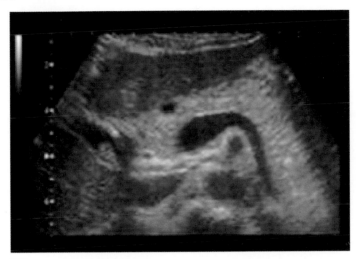

TS pancreas

Q1. What is the diagnosis?

A1. Insulinoma (pancreatic islet cell tumour)

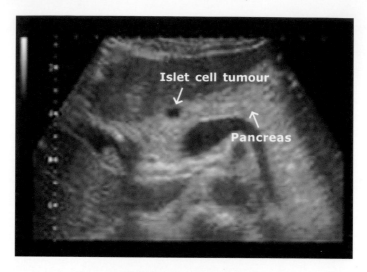

Notes

Insulinoma is a neuroendocrine tumour which arises from pancreatic islet cells. They secrete insulin causing recurrent attacks of hypoglycaemia and the diagnosis is usually suggested from a combination of clinical symptoms and hormonal assays. The role of imaging is to determine the location of the lesion. 90% of cases are benign and surgical resection is usually curative.

Ultrasound Features
- Small (usually < 2 cm), well-defined, echo-poor mass
- Most commonly found in the pancreatic head

Hints

Islet cell tumours are notoriously difficult to locate because of their small size, particularly if they are located in the tail of the gland which is often obscured by bowel gas shadows. Visualisation of this region can be helped by giving the patient a fluid load and using the stomach as an acoustic window.

Other less common islet cell tumours include:
- Gastrinoma – secretes gastrin, causing peptic ulceration
- Glucagonoma – secretes glucagon, causing diabetes
- Non-functioning islet cell tumour – tend to be larger in size and the majority are malignant

CASE 10

A 50-year-old alcoholic man is referred with abdominal pain.

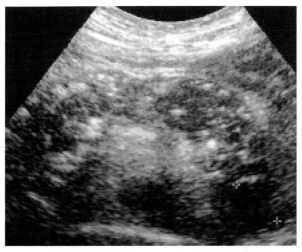

TS pancreas

Q1. What is the diagnosis?
Q2. What is the cystic structure being measured?

A1. Chronic pancreatitis
A2. Pancreatic pseudocyst

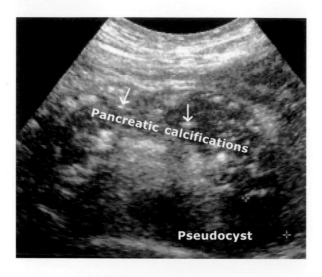

Notes
Chronic pancreatitis is progressive destruction of pancreatic tissue caused by recurrent episodes of mild or sub-clinical pancreatitis. In the vast majority of cases it is alcohol related but can be hereditary or secondary to longstanding ductal obstruction. Patients suffer with recurrent bouts of upper abdominal pain, steatorrhoea or diabetes.

Ultrasound Features
• Small atrophic pancreas
• Speckled pancreatic calcifications
• Dilated pancreatic duct
• Associated pseudocysts

Hints
Other causes of an echo-bright pancreas include:
• Advanced age
• Cystic fibrosis
• Obesity
• Steroids

Scattered glandular calcifications are the hallmark of chronic pancreatitis.

CASE 11

A 58-year-old woman presents with weight loss, nausea and jaundice.

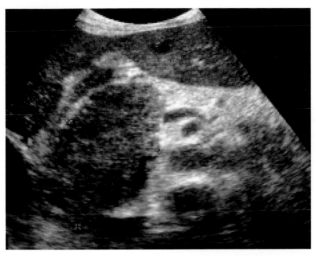

TS pancreas

Q1. What is the diagnosis?

A1. Carcinoma of the head of pancreas

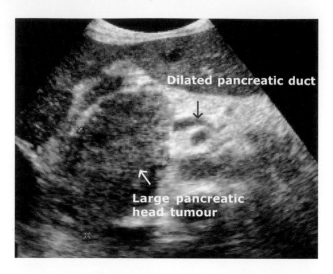

Notes

Pancreatic adenocarcinoma is an aggressive malignancy with a poor prognosis. The majority occur in the pancreatic head where they cause obstructive jaundice and epigastric pain. Less than 10% of cases are suitable for curative surgical resection (Whipple's operation) because of invasion into adjacent vascular structures and distant metastatic disease.

Ultrasound Features
- Echo-poor lesion with irregular margins
- Disruption of normal anatomy
- 'Double duct sign' – dilated pancreatic duct and CBD

Hints

The pancreatic duct is considered dilated if it is >2 mm in diameter.

Imaging signs of unresectability:
- Invasion into adjacent vascular structures, e.g., splenic and portal vein
- Lymph node metastases, e.g., para-aortic
- Distant metastases, e.g., liver, lung, bone

CASE 12

A 40-year-old woman presents with severe epigastric pain and vomiting.

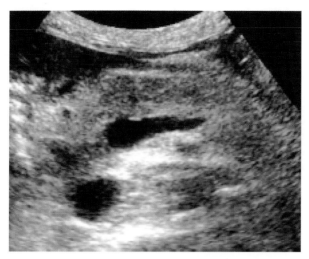

TS pancreas

Q1. What is the diagnosis?
Q2. What is the commonest cause?

A1. Acute pancreatitis
A2. Gallstones

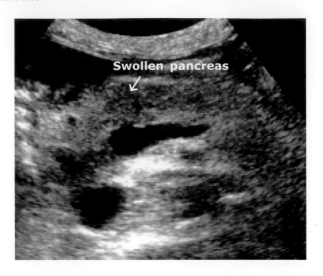

Notes
Acute pancreatitis is inflammation of the pancreas with parenchymal destruction caused by the release of proteolytic enzymes. Patients present with severe epigastric pain and can be moribund from sepsis and multiorgan failure. The majority of cases are caused by gallstone obstruction of the pancreatic duct, but other causes include alcohol, trauma, steroids and autoimmune conditions. Laboratory findings include elevated serum amylase and lipase levels.

Ultrasound Features
- Swollen/enlarged pancreas
- Echo-poor (may be difficult to visualise)
- Tender in the midline
- Fluid in the flanks

Hints
It takes up to 24 hours for the ultrasound changes to appear.

Examine the biliary tree for dilatation and look for an obstructing gallstone in the region of the ampulla of Vater; these patients may benefit from an ERCP with sphincterotomy and stone removal.

Follow-up scans in the weeks after an attack are used to look for complications:

- Splenic/portal vein thrombosis
- Splenic artery pseudoaneurysm
- Pancreatic pseudocyst (echo-poor collection adjacent to the gland)

CASE 13

A 30-year-old man is rushed into A&E unconscious following a high-speed RTA. An ultrasound scan is performed.

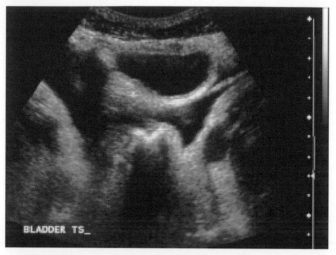

TS Bladder

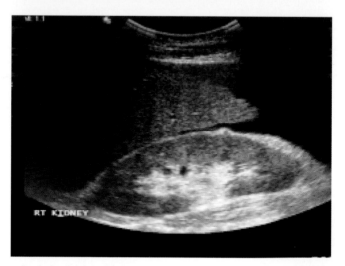

LS right kidney/liver

Q1. What is the diagnosis?
Q2. What is a likely cause?

A1. Haemoperitoneum
A2. Splenic injury

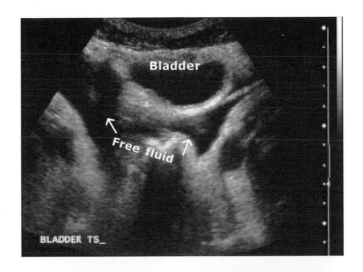

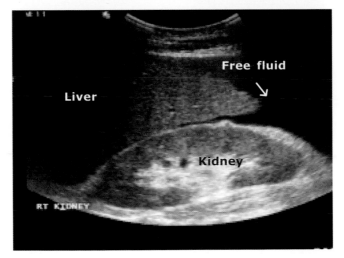

Notes

FAST (Focussed Assessment Sonography of Trauma) scanning is increasingly being used in the emergency department. It employs a 4-view approach for rapid detection of haemoperitoneum and pericardial fluid, which helps direct acute management of the severely injured patient.

Ultrasound Features

Examine the following areas looking for free fluid:
- Pelvis – pelvic fluid
- Left upper quadrant – peri-splenic fluid
- Right upper quadrant – Morrison's pouch fluid
- Substernal (4-chamber cardiac view) – pericardial fluid

Hints

FAST scanning is not indicated for assessment of visceral organ injury such as splenic/liver lacerations (CT remains the modality of choice for these). However, it has a role to play in acute assessment of the trauma patient.

Splenic injury is the most common cause of haemoperitoneum in blunt abdominal trauma. Scanning the spleen in these cases may reveal disruption of normal splenic contour, intraparenchymal haemorrhage (echo-bright area) or peri-splenic haematoma (echo-poor collection).

CASE 14

A 20-year-old man presents with sore throat, fever, general malaise and upper abdominal discomfort.

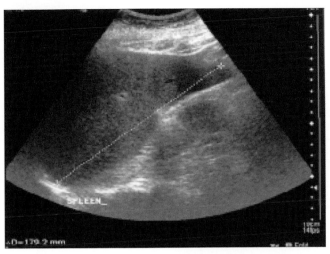

LS spleen

Q1. What is the diagnosis?
Q2. What is the likely cause?

A1. Moderate splenomegaly
A2. Infectious mononucleosis

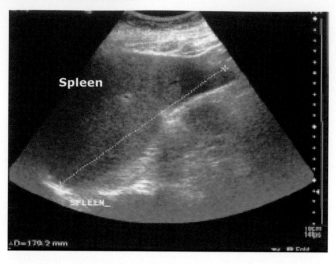

Notes

There are many causes of splenomegaly, but the commonest causes of mild–moderate enlargement as in this case are portal hypertension, lymphoma, infectious mononucleosis and haemolytic anaemia. Review of clinical history is essential.

Splenomegaly is considered to be 'massive' when it requires extended field of view imaging to be measured. Common causes of massive enlargement are chronic myeloid leukaemia, myelofibrosis and malaria.

Ultrasound Features

• >13 cm measuring from inferior pole to superior pole.
• Inferior margin becomes rounded.

Hints

To aid splenic assessment ask the patient to place their left arm behind their head; this will widen the intercostal space and increase the scan 'window'.

Look for clues as to the cause:
?cirrhotic liver, ascites – suggests portal hypertension
?focal lesions in spleen – suggests lymphoma or metastases
?hepatomegaly or lymphadenopathy – suggests lymphoma

Splenomegaly in association with infectious mononucleosis will reverse with time, taking around 2–3 months to return to normal size. A well recognised complication is splenic rupture following minimal trauma.

Chapter 3

Liver and Liver Transplant

CASE 1

A 65-year-old man with COPD is referred for abdominal ultrasound because of mildly abnormal liver function tests.

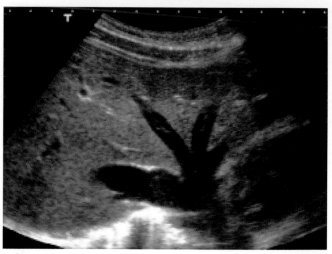

TS hepatic veins

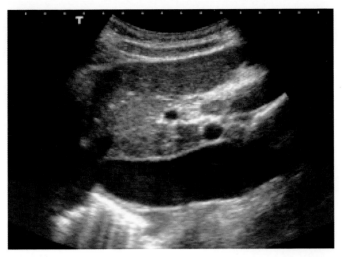

LS IVC

Q1. What are the findings?
Q2. What is the likely diagnosis?

A1. Dilated IVC and hepatic veins
A2. Liver congestion caused by right heart failure

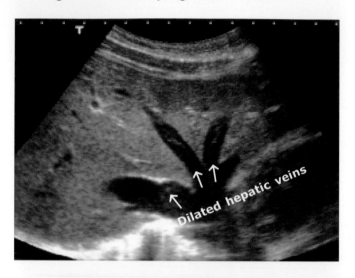

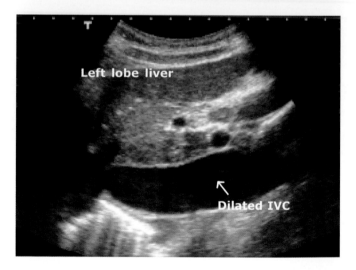

Notes

The commonest causes of right heart dysfunction are ischaemia and chronic obstructive pulmonary disease. Transmitted back pressure into the hepatic veins causes hepatic congestion and liver enzyme abnormalities. If severe and long standing, it can cause cirrhosis (cardiac cirrhosis).

Ultrasound Features
- Dilated hepatic veins
- Dilated IVC (>2 cm AP diameter)
- Giant 'a' waves with hepatic vein Doppler

Hints
The hepatic vein Doppler 'a' wave represents transmitted back pressure during atrial systole. Normally there is some blood flow towards the probe during this phase of the cardiac cycle; however, large-volume flow indicates right heart dysfunction (tricuspid regurgitation).

CASE 2

A 40-year-old man who is a heavy drinker is referred for abdominal ultrasound.

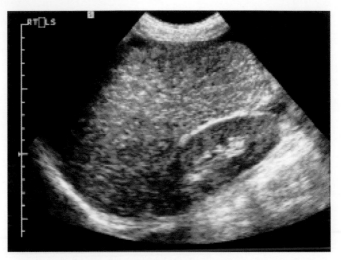

LS right kidney/liver

Q1. What is the diagnosis?

A1. Cirrhosis

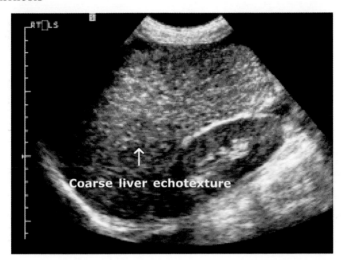

Notes

Cirrhosis is a chronic disease of the liver characterised by extensive collagen deposition with periportal and bridging fibrosis. There is distortion of the normal hepatic lobular architecture with areas of nodular regeneration. In late-stage disease there is a generalised reduction of liver volume with atrophy of the right lobe, and prominence of the left and caudate lobes. Portal hypertension develops secondary to increased resistance within an abnormally 'stiff' liver. Alcohol and chronic hepatitis B and C infection account for the majority of cases. Cirrhosis is a major risk factor for developing hepatocellular carcinoma.

Ultrasound Features
- Small contracted liver
- Irregular and nodular surface
- Coarse parenchymal echotexture
- Loss of respiratory variation in portal vein waveform

Hints
Look for other signs of portal hypertension:
- Ascites
- Splenomegaly
- Gastric/splenic varices

CASE 3

A 45-year-old man with alcoholic liver disease is admitted following several episodes of haematemesis.

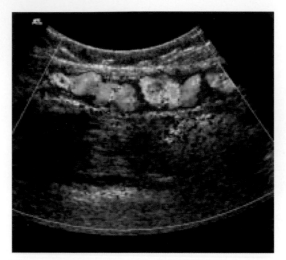

TS umbilicus

Q1. What is this abnormal vessel?
Q2. What is the diagnosis?

A1. Recanalised umbilical vein
A2. Portal hypertension

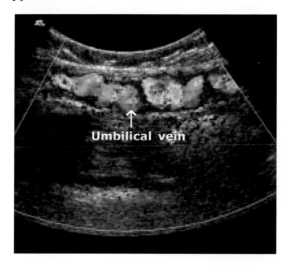

Notes

In advanced stage cirrhosis with portal hypertension, the liver is 'stiff' and offers increased resistance to forward venous flow. As a result, portosystemic collateral channels develop which redirect blood into lowpressure systemic vessels. One of these pathways involves the umbilical vein – a communication between the portal vein and the anterior abdominal wall veins. Treatment options for portal hypertension include endoscopic injection sclerotherapy and transjugular intrahepatic portosystemic shunt (TIPSS) placement.

Ultrasound Features

- Cirrhotic liver
- Common portosystemic collaterals:

Gastric varices: tortuous veins in the midline around the stomach
Splenic varices: tortuous veins at the splenic hilum
Gallbladder varices: tortuous veins within a thickened gallbladder wall
Recanalised umbilical vein: between left portal vein and anterior abdominal wall

Hints

Look for other signs of portal hypertension:

- Abnormal portal vein blood flow
- Ascites
- Splenomegaly (can be normal due to portosystemic decompression)

CASE 4

A 40-year-old man who had an orthotopic liver transplant 4 days ago has rising transaminase levels.

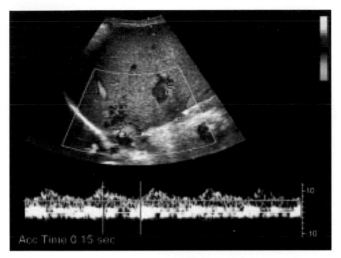

Hepatic artery spectral Doppler

Q1. What does this Doppler waveform demonstrate?
Q2. What is the diagnosis?

A1. Parvus tardus waveform
A2. Hepatic artery stenosis

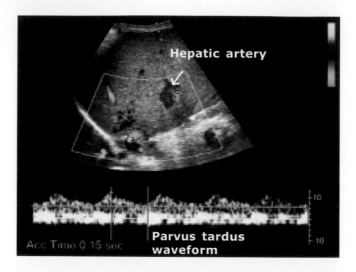

Notes
Hepatic artery stenosis occurs in around 10% of transplant recipients, and is most common at the anastomotic site as a result of arterial clamp injury. Most patients present within the first few weeks with deteriorating liver function tests. Untreated it leads to biliary ischaemia with hepatic dysfunction and there is a high risk of progression to hepatic artery thrombosis. Arterial thrombosis is a surgical emergency as the hepatic artery is the sole provider of oxygenation for the biliary system.

Ultrasound Features
- Parvus tardus hepatic artery Doppler waveform
- Prolonged acceleration time (>0.08 sec)

Hints
In the first 48 hours following a transplant it is normal to just see a small systolic spike with minimal or absent end-diastolic flow. Any waveform abnormality beyond 48 hours merits frequent re-examination.

CASE 5

A 65-year-old man who was recently discharged following an episode of cholecystitis is systemically unwell with fever, rigors and abdominal pain.

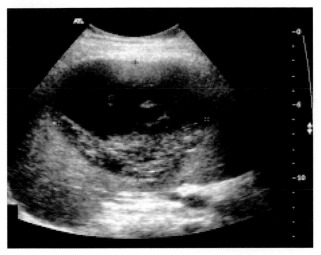

TS right lobe liver

Q1. What is the diagnosis?

A1. Liver abscess

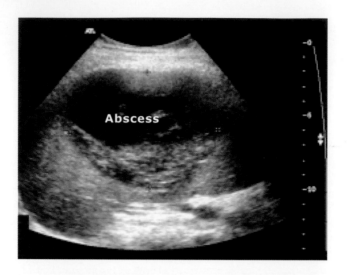

Notes

The majority of liver abscesses in the western world are pyogenic and caused by ascending biliary tree infection. Other sources include gastrointestinal infections and disseminated sepsis (e.g., endocarditis). *E. coli* is the commonest bacteria, but other anaerobic and aerobic organisms can be involved. Amoebic abscesses are common in India, Africa and the Far East. The mortality from a liver abscess is high and prompt drainage is required, either surgically or via radiologically-guided techniques.

Ultrasound Features

- Echo-poor lesion with an irregular wall
- Contains 'lumpy' echo-bright debris
- Display variable post-acoustic enhancement
- Intense reverberation artifacts seen with gas-forming organisms

Hints

Multiple hepatic microabscesses can be seen in association with disseminated fungal disease. Patients are severely immunosuppressed, often with haematologic malignancies, and candida albicans is the commonest pathogen. Fungal micro-abscesses may also involve the spleen and occasionally the kidney. They appear as multiple small echo-poor nodules with a central echo-bright nidus.

CASE 6

A 28-year-old woman is referred for an abdominal ultrasound by her GP for investigation of hepatomegaly.

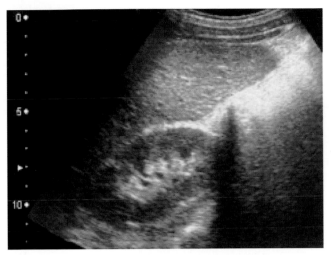

LS right lobe

Q1. What is the diagnosis?

A1. Riedel's lobe

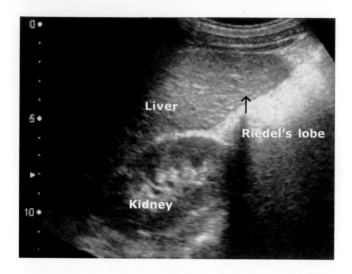

Notes

Riedel's lobe is a tongue-like projection from the inferior surface of the right lobe of liver. It is a common anatomical variant and of no clinical significance. Rarely it may extend down as far as the right iliac fossa.

Ultrasound Features

- Segment 6 of the liver extends below inferior pole of the right kidney.
- Segment 6 has a 'pointed margin'.
- Left lobe of liver tends to be smaller than normal.

Hints

Distinguish from true hepatomegaly:
- Segment 6 has a 'rounded margin'.
- Both right and left lobes are usually enlarged.

CASE 7

A 40-year-old type 2 diabetic is referred by her GP after blood tests showed mildly raised transaminase levels. She is asymptomatic.

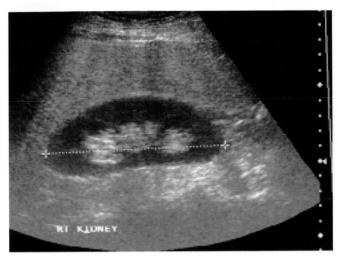

LS right kidney/liver

Q1. What is the diagnosis?

A1. Hepatic steatosis (fatty liver)

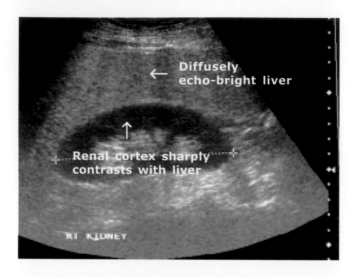

Notes

Fatty infiltration of the liver is caused by increased deposition of triglycerides. It occurs in various conditions including diabetes, chronic alcoholism, pregnancy, parenteral nutrition and cystic fibrosis. Steatosis can be focal or diffuse. Most patients are asymptomatic, but liver function tests may be mildly deranged.

Ultrasound Features

- Mild hepatomegaly.
- Liver echogenicity is much brighter than adjacent renal cortex.
- Loss of portal vein wall definition.
- Post attenuation fall out.

Hints

The parenchymal changes in fatty liver make small focal liver lesions difficult to detect and this should be indicated on the report.

Other causes of an echo-bright liver include chronic hepatitis and cirrhosis.

Causes of an echo-poor liver include acute hepatitis and leukaemic infiltration.

CASE 8

A 50-year-old man known to have hepatitis B – induced chronic liver disease is referred with weight loss and worsening ascites.

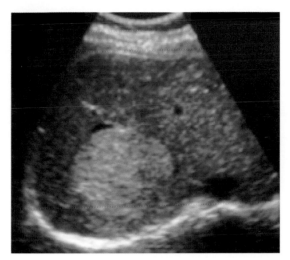

TS right lobe liver

Q1. What is the diagnosis?

A1. Hepatocellular carcinoma

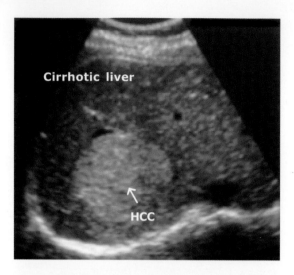

Notes
Hepatocellular carcinoma is the commonest abdominal malignancy worldwide. It usually occurs as a complication of chronic liver disease, most often in patients with cirrhosis. Imaging appearances are non-specific and when combined with a disorganised background parenchyma this makes diagnosis challenging. Vascular invasion with portal or hepatic venous thrombosis is a very suggestive finding and indicates advanced stage disease.

Ultrasound Features
- Variable echo-pattern depending upon fibrous tissue and fat content.
- Small tumours are typically echo-poor.
- Larger tumours are typically echo-bright (fat and haemorrhage).

Hints
Look for indirect evidence of tumour, e.g., localised surface bulge.

Examine the portal and hepatic veins for tumour thrombus.

Hepatocellular carcinoma can be diffusely infiltrating giving a generalised echotexture abnormality.

CASE 9

A 45-year-old woman who is on total parenteral nutrition for Crohn's disease is having an abdominal ultrasound.

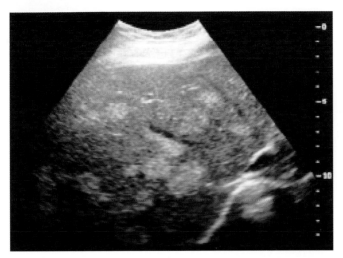

TS right lobe liver

Q1. What is the diagnosis?

A1. Focal fatty infiltration

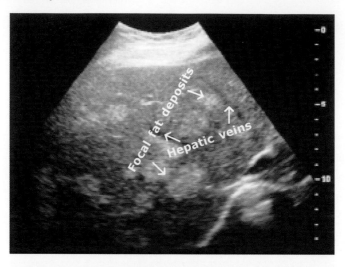

Notes

Hepatic steatosis can be diffuse or focal. Focal fat deposition usually has a characteristic 'fan shaped' appearance extending to the liver edge, but it can have a nodular and multifocal appearance simulating echo-bright metastases. The absence of mass effect with non-distorted traversing blood vessels is a key distinguishing feature in such cases.

Ultrasound Features

- Focal echo-bright areas.
- Angulated margin.
- The most characteristic location is the peri-hilar region.

Hints

Clinical correlation is essential in these cases. If there is any doubt as to the diagnosis, further imaging is required. MRI easily distinguishes fat from more sinister pathology.

CASE 10

A 22-year-old man with a chronic lung disease is having an annual abdominal ultrasound assessment.

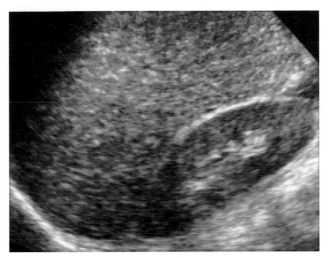

LS right lobe liver

Q1. What does this image show?
Q2. What is the unifying diagnosis?

A1. Focal areas of biliary cirrhosis
A2. Cystic fibrosis

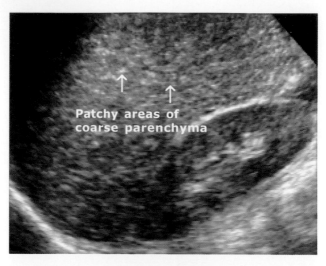

Notes

Cystic fibrosis is a common inherited disease with autosomal recessive pattern of transmission. It results in abnormally viscous secretions which cause well-known pulmonary manifestations of bronchiectasis and recurrent infections. More patients are now surviving into adulthood and extrapulmonary manifestations are increasingly being detected. Liver disease is the second leading cause of death in cystic fibrosis. Viscous secretions cause biliary stasis and inflammatory reaction with peri-ductal fibrosis. Focal biliary cirrhosis is a characteristic pathological finding and seen in up to 80% of patients. A small percentage progress to multinodular cirhhosis.

Ultrasound Features
- Echo-bright peri-portal thickening
- Patchy areas of coarse parenchyma
- Fatty infiltration

Hints

Other abdominal ultrasound findings in cystic fibrosis include:
- Hepatic steatosis
- Fatty replacement of the pancreas and chronic pancreatitis
- Gallstones, ductal strictures and microgallbladder

CASE 11

A 50-year-old man with weight loss and altered bowel habit is referred for an abdominal ultrasound.

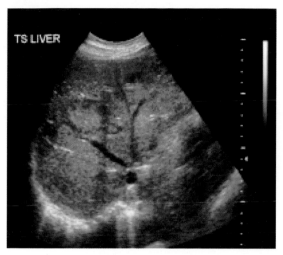

TS right lobe liver

Q1. What does this image show?
Q2. What is the likely cause?

A1. Liver metastasis
A2. Colorectal carcinoma

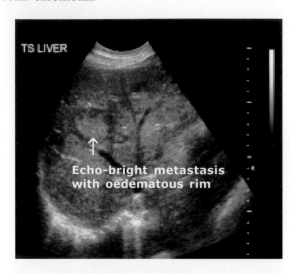

Notes
The liver is a common site of metastatic disease because of its rich blood supply and sinusoidal anatomy which traps small clusters of cells. Colorectal carcinoma is the commonest metastatic cancer to occur in the liver. Other primary tumours which commonly metastasize to the liver include stomach, pancreas, lung and breast. Partial hepatic resection is an established treatment option for colorectal metastases confined to the liver.

Ultrasound Features
• Wide variation in appearance
• Typically an echo-bright lesion with a rim of oedema – 'target appearance'
• Exhibit mass effect with distortion of traversing blood vessels
• May be single or multiple, cystic or solid

Hints
Diagnostic dilemmas can occur with benign lesions such as focal fatty infiltration, focal nodular hyperplasia and haemangiomas.

Microbubble contrast agents aid further characterisation of these lesions by providing information regarding their vascular supply.

CASE 12

A 25-year-old woman who had an orthotopic liver transplant 12 months ago presents with fevers, weight loss and vague abdominal discomfort.

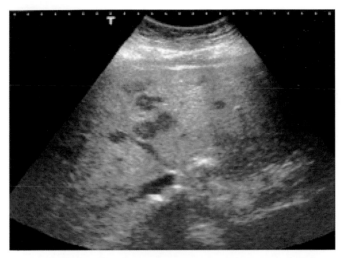

TS right lobe liver

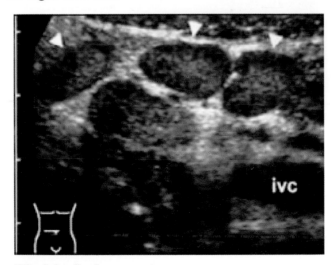

TS right flank

Q1. What do these images show?
Q2. What is the diagnosis?

A1. Multiple intrahepatic masses
Nodal mass at the porta hepatis
A2. Post Transplant Lymphoproliferative disorder

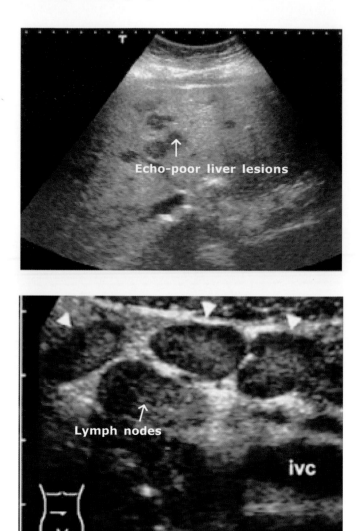

Notes

Post transplant lymphoproliferative disorder (PTLD) is an unusual complication in adults (1–2%) but affects up to 10% of paediatric liver transplant patients. PTLD represents a spectrum of disorders from benign reactive nodal enlargement through to full-blown malignant B cell lymphoma. It is associated with high-dose immunosuppressive therapy and may be associated with Epstein-Barr virus. PTLD typically occurs between 6 and 18 months post transplantation and one of the characteristic features is the high incidence of extra-nodal disease.

Ultrasound Features

- Single or multiple echo-poor liver masses
- Masses may also be seen in kidneys, bowel and spleen
- Multiple sites of abdominal lymphadenopathy

Hints

The differential diagnosis of multiple parenchymal lesions in the transplanted liver is wide and includes abscesses, metastases and PTLD. Clinical presentation helps narrow the differential diagnosis but histo-pathological analysis is ultimately required.

Treatment of PTLD involves reduction/cessation of immuno-suppressive drugs and interferon-α is also sometimes used. Despite this, mortality is around 70%.

CASE 13

A 40-year-old woman with weight loss is having a routine abdominal ultrasound.

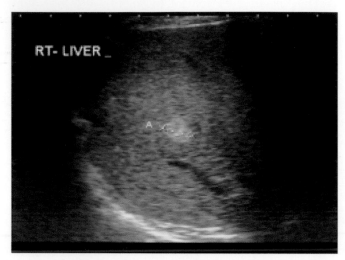

LS right lobe liver

Q1. What is this liver lesion?

A1. Haemangioma

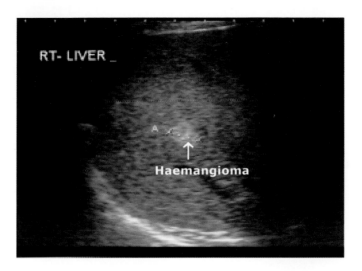

Notes
Haemangiomas are the commonest benign hepatic tumours affecting up to 20% of adults. The majority are clinically silent and they are common incidental findings. Histologically they consist of multiple vascular channels with a single layer of endothelial cells. They appear avascular with colour Doppler imaging as blood is slow flowing within them.

Ultrasound Features
- Small, well-defined, echo-bright lesion.
- Usually solitary and in a peripheral location.
- Post-acoustic enhancement is common.

Hints
In the clinical context of an asymptomatic patient with no history of malignant disease the above 'typical' ultrasound appearance is diagnostic. However, up to 30% of haemangiomas have atypical ultrasound features. They can appear uniformly echo-poor, contain cystic areas or have a very heterogeneous echo-texture. Such appearances create diagnostic confusion and MRI may be required for definitive lesion characterisation.

CASE 14

A 60-year-old man with polycythaemia rubra vera presents with abdominal pain, distension and raised liver enzymes.

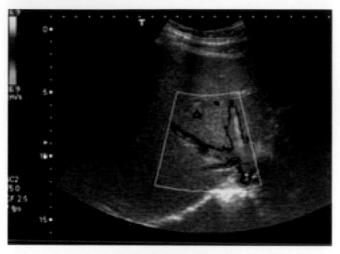

TS hepatic veins with colour Doppler

Q1. What is the diagnosis?

A1. Acute Budd-Chiari syndrome

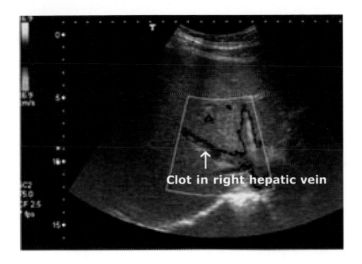

Notes

Budd-Chiari syndrome is obstruction of hepatic venous outflow which may be idiopathic or associated with underlying disease. Causes include hypercoagulable states, pregnancy, obstructing tumour thrombus and congenita fibrous webs of the inferior vena cava. Patients present acutely with hepatomegaly, ascites and liver dysfunction. In longstanding cases the liver becomes atrophic, but the caudate lobe is preserved as it drains directly into the inferior vena cava.

Ultrasound Features
Acute
- Hepatomegaly
- Ascites
- Reversed or absent flow in hepatic veins
- May see thrombus in hepatic veins/IVC

Chronic
- Small atrophic liver with normal caudate lobe
- Intra-hepatic vein-vein shunts
- Splenomegaly

Hints

Radiologically placed hepatic vein stents are increasingly used as an alternative to surgical portosystemic shunting in these cases.

Chapter 4

Gynaecology

CASE 1

A 62-year-old woman is referred with abdominal pain and distension.

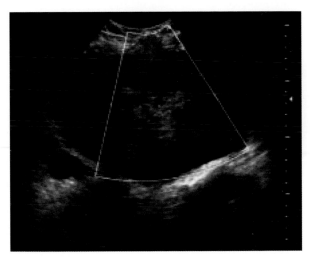

TS right adnexa

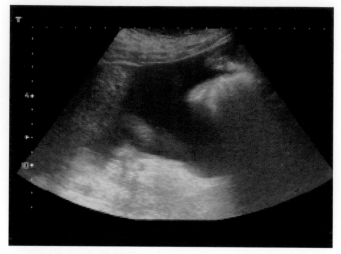

TS left paraumbilical

Q1. What is the diagnosis?
Q2. What does image 2 indicate?

A1. Ovarian carcinoma
A2. Omental disease and ascites

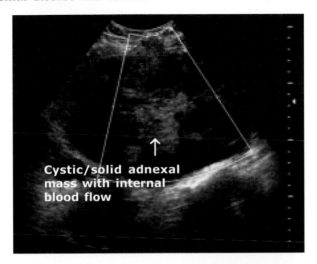

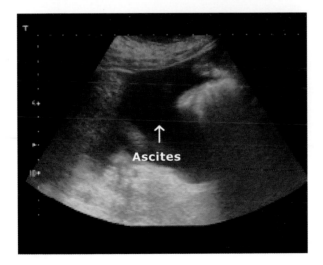

Notes
Ovarian carcinoma is a common gynaecological malignancy with a peak incidence in the 6th decade. Risk factors include nulliparity, early menarche, late menopause and family history. Onset is insidious with few early symptoms and most patients have advanced disease at time of presentation.

There are many histological subtypes of which serous and mucinous cystadenocarcinomas are the commonest. Ultrasound, MRI and CT have complimentary roles in the staging of these tumours.

Ultrasound Features
Cystic adnexal mass with malignant features:
- Thick irregular walls
- Thick internal septations
- Internal echoes
- Internal blood flow
- Papillary wall nodules

Hints
Always examine the rest of the abdomen for signs of advanced disease:
- Omental thickening
- Ascites
- Liver surface metastases
- Pleural effusions
- Hydronephrosis (ureteric obstruction)

CASE 2

A 58-year-old woman is referred with post-menopausal bleeding. She was diagnosed with breast cancer 12 months ago.

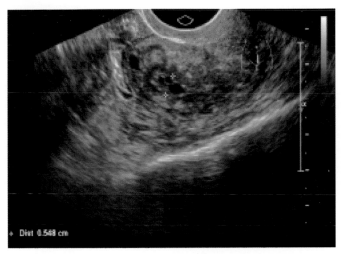

LS uterus

Q1. What is the diagnosis?
Q2. What is the cause of this appearance?

A1. Cystic endometrial hyperplasia
A2. Tamoxifen

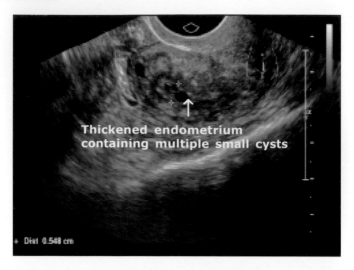

Notes
Tamoxifen is an anti-oestrogen drug prescribed for both pre- and post-menopausal women with breast cancer. It has been shown to increase survival. The majority of patients taking it develop endometrial changes which become visible with ultrasound within 12 months.

Ultrasound Features
- Endometrial hyperplasia with small cystic spaces
- Endometrial polyps (30%)
- Endometrial carcinoma (x6 risk)

Hints
In post-menopausal women a normal endometrial thickness is <5 mm.

The average thickness for a patient taking tamoxifen is around 10 mm.

Thickening greater than this or thickening associated with post-menopausal bleeding requires referral for hysteroscopy +/– biopsy.

CASE 3

A 30-year-old woman is referred with pelvic pain, fever and raised inflammatory markers.

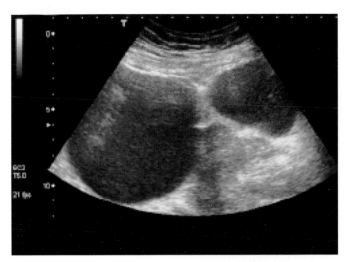

TS right adnexa

Q1. What is the diagnosis?

A1. Tubo-ovarian abscess

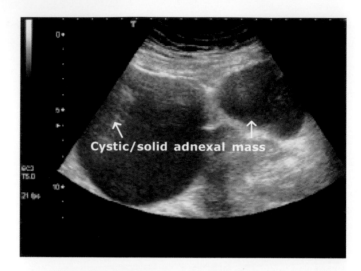

Notes

Tubo-ovarian abscess is a late complication of pelvic inflammatory disease. Pus from the fallopian tube becomes walled off by pelvic adhesions and inflammatory reaction involves the ovary, broad ligaments and adjacent bowel. Patients present with pelvic pain and fever.

Ultrasound Features
- Septated cystic adnexal mass containing debris
- Adnexal tenderness
- Free fluid in the pouch of Douglas

Hints

There are many causes of a complex adnexal mass and clinical correlation is essential. Differential diagnosis includes:
- Haemorrhagic ovarian cyst
- Appendix abscess
- Ovarian carcinoma
- Ectopic pregnancy
- Crohn's abscess

CASE 4

A 25-year-old woman has attended for investigation of menorrhagia.

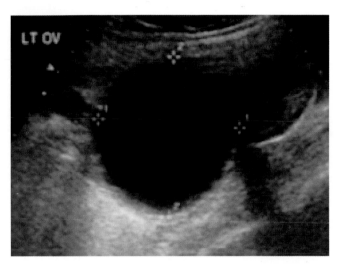

TS left adnexa

Q1. What does this image show?

A1. Simple ovarian cyst

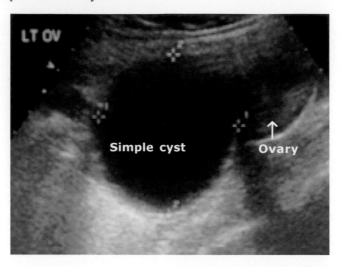

Notes

Simple cysts such as this are common incidental findings. The majority are follicular cysts which occur when the dominant (graafian) follicle fails to rupture.

Ultrasound Features
- Smooth edge
- Thin wall
- Echo-free contents
- Post-acoustic enhancement

Hints

Simple cysts <3 cm in a pre-menopausal or <5 cm in a post-menopausal woman are of no clinical significance and do not need to be followed up.

Larger cysts or those with atypical features require a repeat scan in 6–8 weeks time to check for size reduction/resolution.

CASE 5

A 55-year-old woman presents with post-menopausal bleeding. She is taking tamoxifen for breast cancer.

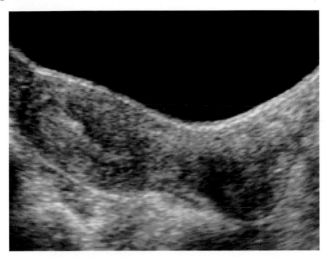

LS uterus

Q1. What is the diagnosis?

A1. Endometrial polyp

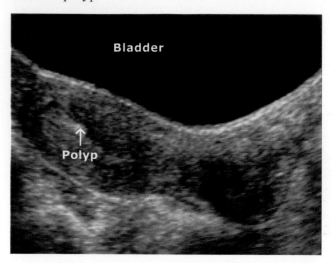

Notes

Polyps are focal areas of endometrial hyperplasia which project into the uterine cavity. There is an association with tamoxifen therapy (up to 30% develop them). They are a common incidental finding but occasionally present with bleeding; rarely they can transform into endometrial carcinoma.

Ultrasound Features

- Focal increase in endometrial thickness.
- Can be single or multiple.
- Usually <1 cm.
- A 'feeding' vessel may be seen entering its base.

Hints

The main differential diagnosis is a submucosal fibroid. Polyps will have the same echogenicity as adjacent endometrium whereas fibroids are usually more echo-poor.

Sonohysterography is useful to confirm the diagnosis. This involves instillation of normal saline into the uterine cavity while scanning and outlines polyps more clearly.

CASE 6

A 30-year-old woman presents with sudden-onset left-sided lower abdominal pain.

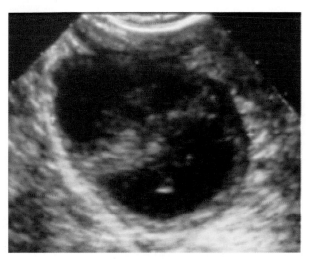

TS left adnexa

Q1. What is the diagnosis?

A1. Haemorrhagic ovarian cyst

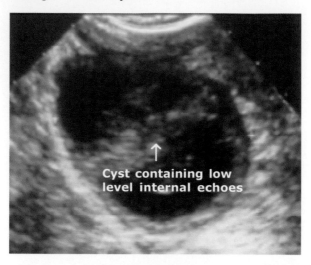

Cyst containing low level internal echoes

Notes

Spontaneous haemorrhage can occur into any ovarian cyst, but is particularly common with the corpus luteal type. These cysts occur when the dominant (graafian) follicle fails to involute following ovulation. Cyst haemorrhage typically causes sudden-onset pelvic pain and tenderness on the affected side. The main complication is cyst rupture with haemoperitoneum and hypovolaemic shock.

Ultrasound Features
- Adnexal tenderness
- Complex cystic adnexal mass
- Free fluid in the pouch of Douglas with cyst rupture

Hints

The main differential diagnoses are ectopic pregnancy and ovarian torsion.

Torsion results from twisting of the ovary on its vascular pedicle leading to congestion and infarction. Ovarian cysts predispose to torsion by acting as a fulcrum. The affected ovary is enlarged and oedematous with peripheral dilated follicles.

CASE 7

A 33-year-old woman is referred with menorrhagia.

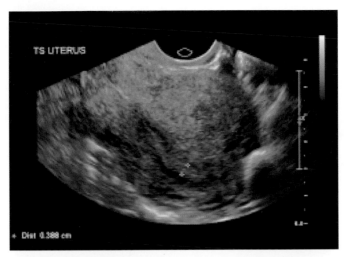

LS uterus

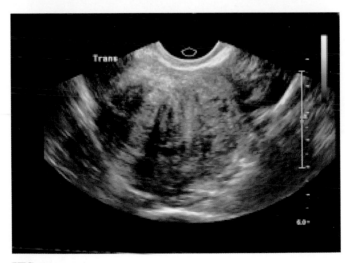

ITS uterus

Q1. What is the diagnosis?

A1. Fibroids (leiomyoma)

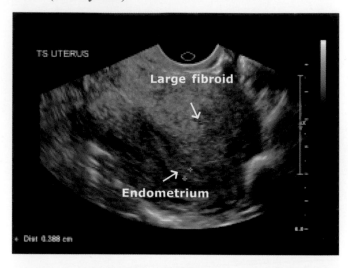

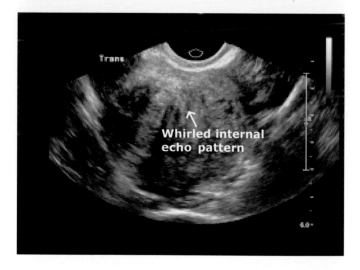

Notes

These are a very common finding (25% of pre-menopausal women). Fibroids are benign smooth muscle tumours with a fibrous element. They are oestrogen dependant, growing during pregnancy, with a tendency to regress after the menopause. Most are asymptomatic, but they can cause menorrhagia, pain or subfertility, depending on their size and location.

Ultrasound Features

- Focal uterine enlargement.
- Well-defined echo-poor mass with lamellated/whirled internal echo pattern.
- May contain echo-bright areas of calcification.
- Doppler shows circumferential fibroidal blood vessels.

Hints

Rapidly enlarging fibroids can outgrow their blood supply resulting in painful infarction. Such degenerating fibroids can have a very bizarre ultrasound appearance including large central cystic areas.

A large fibroidal uterus can exert pressure effects on the bladder causing frequency of micturition and occasionally ureteric obstruction. Always complete a gynaecological ultrasound examination by imaging both kidneys.

CASE 8

A 67-year-old woman is referred for investigation of post-menopausal bleeding.

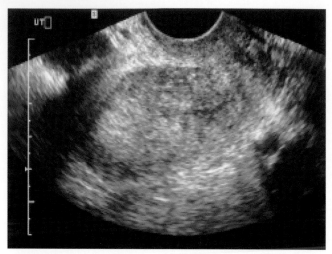

LS uterus

Q1. What is the diagnosis?

A1. Endometrial carcinoma

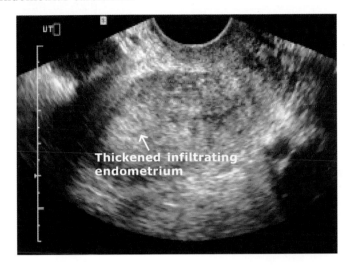

Notes
Endometrial carcinoma is primarily a disease of post-menopausal women with a peak age of 60 years. It can arise from endometrial hyperplasia or occur de novo. Risk factors include nulliparity, late menopause and tamoxifen therapy. Patients present with post-menopausal bleeding.

Ultrasound Features
- Thickened endometrium with irregular margins
- Endometrial mass of mixed echogenicity
- Endometrial mass seen infiltrating into the myometrium
- Strong intra-tumoral blood flow

Hints
The endometrium is considered thickened if >15 mm in a pre-menopausal woman and >5 mm in a post-menopausal woman.

Ultrasound cannot reliably distinguish between hyperplasia and carcinoma and hysteroscopy +/- biopsy is required in all cases.

MRI is the modality of choice for assessing myometrial invasion.

CASE 9

A 25-year-old woman is referred for investigation of infertility.

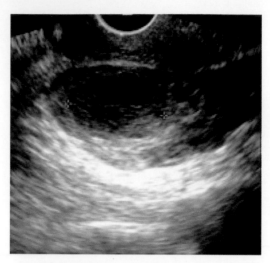

TS right adnexa

Q1. What is the diagnosis?

A1. Endometrioma

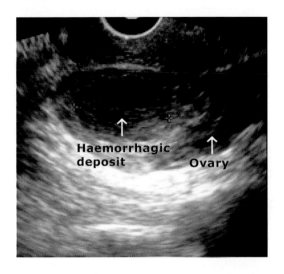

Notes

Endometriosis is a common condition affecting 5% of all women. Endometrial tissue implants outside the uterine cavity and undergoes cyclical changes with haemorrhage, inflammation and formation of adhesions. It presents with pelvic pain and infertility. Common sites include the ovaries (80%), pouch of Douglas and the uterosacral ligaments. Other sites include the serosal surface of the colon, bladder and rarely the pleura.

Ultrasound Features
• Ovarian cyst containing low-level internal echoes (blood)

Hints
The sometimes complex appearance of an endometrioma can mimic:
• Haemorrhagic ovarian cyst
• Tubo-ovarian abscess
• Ovarian neoplasm

MRI is the modality of choice for imaging endometriosis elsewhere in the abdomen and pelvis.

Indirect evidence of pelvic/bowel adhesions may be seen using the visceral slide assessment – lack of free movement of the pelvic organs with deep respiration and manual palpation.

CASE 10

A 35-year-old woman presents with abdominal pain and vomiting.

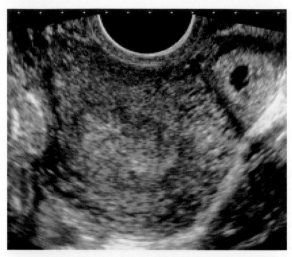

TS uterus

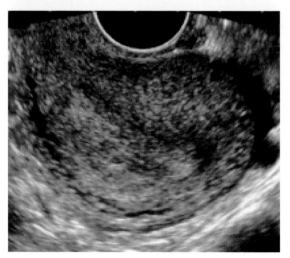

LS uterus

Q1. What is the diagnosis?

A1. Ectopic pregnancy

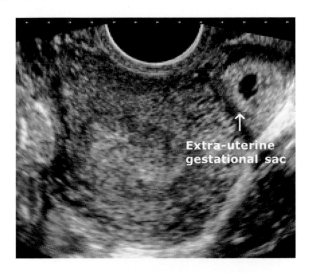

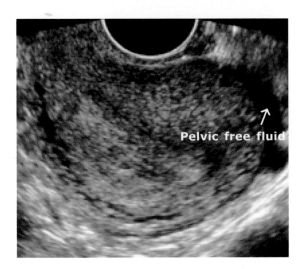

Notes

Ectopic pregnancy is implantation outside the endometrial cavity. The majority are located in the fallopian tubes. Risk factors include prior ectopic, past history of pelvic inflammatory disease, tubal surgery and in vitro fertilization. Patients have a positive pregnancy test and present with vaginal bleeding, abdominal pain and sometimes collapse/hypovolaemic shock if ruptured.

Ultrasound Features

- Demonstration of an extrauterine heartbeat is diagnostic (a rare finding).
- Free fluid (haemoperitoneum) in the pouch of Douglas.
- Echo-bright endometrial thickening from hormonal stimulation.
- A pseudogestational sac is seen in 20%.
- A solid/cystic adnexal mass may be seen.

Hints

Causes of an empty uterus and positive pregnancy test:

- Ectopic pregnancy
- Normal pregnancy <5 weeks
- Miscarriage

As a rule an embryo should always be visible if ß-HCG >1,000 IU.

If an intrauterine pregnancy is found, an ectopic is virtually excluded.

A normal TV scan does not exclude an ectopic pregnancy.

CASE 11

A 25-year-old woman who is 10 weeks pregnant is referred with vaginal bleeding and hyperemesis.

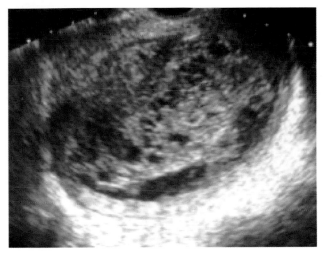

LS uterus

Q1. What is the diagnosis?

A1. Hydatidiform mole

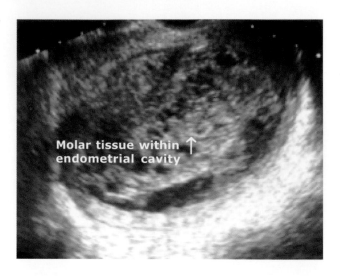

Molar tissue within ↑
endometrial cavity

Notes

Hydatidiform mole is a rare but important condition which occurs in early pregnancy. It occurs when trophoblastic tissue in the placenta undergoes excessive proliferation. Occasionally, fetal tissue forms, but this is nonviable. Patients present with first trimester bleeding and hyperemesis caused by very elevated ß-HCG levels.

Ultrasound Features
- Early stage: enlarged uterus filled with echo-bright material 'snowstorm'
- Later stage: cystic spaces develop within it, 'bunch of grapes'
- Large ovarian theca lutein cysts (excessive ß-HCG stimulation)

Hints

Treatment involves referral to a specialist centre for evacuation of uterine contents and serial monitoring of ß-HCG levels to ensure complete regression.

Approximately 10% develop an invasive mole or malignant choriocarcinoma which is seen as a focal echo-bright lesion invading into the myometrium.

CASE 12

A 28-year-old woman is referred because of secondary amenorrhoea.

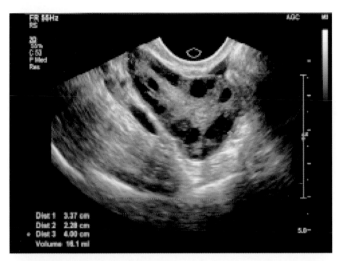

LS right adnexa

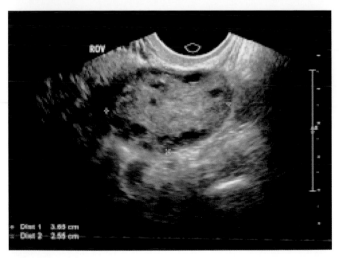

TS right adnexa

Q1. What is the diagnosis?

A1. Polycystic ovarian syndrome

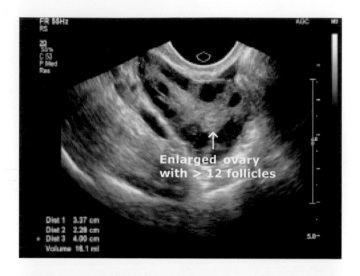

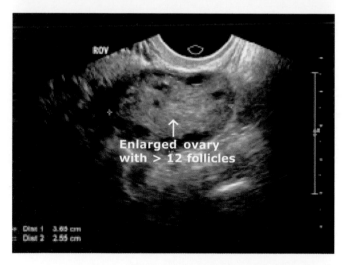

Notes

The polycystic ovarian syndrome (PCOS) is diagnosed on the basis of clinical, biochemical and ultrasound findings. Only about 50% of PCOS patients will have the typical ultrasound findings. The absence of these therefore does not preclude the diagnosis. Patients present with secondary amenorrhoea, weight gain and hirsutism.

Ultrasound Features
- Ovarian volume >10 cm^3
- >12 follicles in an ovary in any one imaging plane.
- Peripheral ovarian stroma is echo-bright.
- Peripheral ovarian stroma is of increased volume.

Hints
PCOS is not to be confused with multicystic ovaries which are seen at the menarche and in anorexia (normal ovarian volumes, less numerous and larger follicles).

Chapter 5

Paediatrics

CASE 1

A 12-year-old girl presents with acute right iliac fossa pain and low-grade fever.

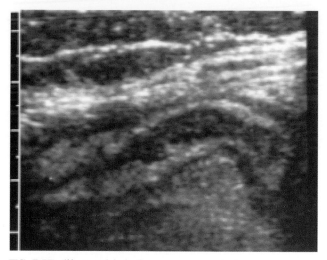

TS RIF (linear high-frequency probe)

Q1. What is the diagnosis?

A1. Acute appendicitis

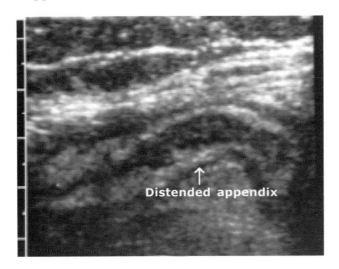

Notes

Appendicitis is the most common cause of an acute surgical abdomen. Obstruction of the appendix lumen leads to mural ischaemia and secondary bacterial infection. Up to 30% of patients present with atypical clinical features and imaging may be helpful to confirm the diagnosis or establish an alternative cause for patient symptoms. Graded compression ultrasound of the right iliac fossa has a high diagnostic accuracy and should be the first-line imaging test in children and women of childbearing age.

Ultrasound Features
- Non-compressible blind-ending tube at the site of maximum tenderness
- Transverse appendix diameter >6 mm
- Hypervascular appendiceal wall

Supportive Features
- Intraluminal faecolith
- Echo-bright peri-appendiceal fat

Hints

Failure to visualise the appendix has been shown to have a strong negative predictive value for appendicitis.

The remainder of the abdomen and pelvis should be routinely examined for 'mimics' of appendicitis such as adnexal, renal and biliary tract pathology.

The acutely inflamed appendix may occasionally be sited in the right upper quadrant, in the midline or to the left of the bladder.

An echo-poor fluid collection (abscess) may be seen in the right flank/pelvis in cases of delayed presentation – caused by appendiceal perforation.

CASE 2

A 4-week-old infant presents with projectile non-bilious vomiting after feeds.

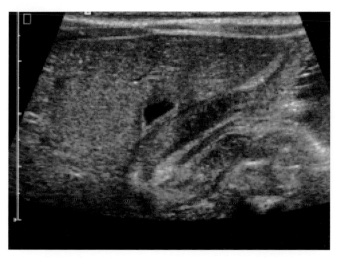

TS epigastrium

Q1. What is the diagnosis?

A1. Hypertrophic pyloric stenosis

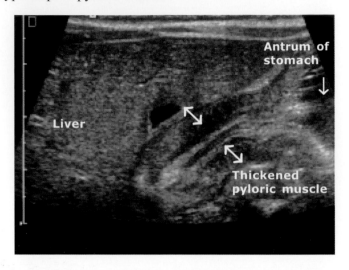

Notes

Hypertrophic pyloric stenosis is caused by hypertrophy of the circular musculature and presents with severe persistent vomiting, a hypochloraemic alkalosis and dehydration in the first few weeks of life. Males are more commonly affected and there is a genetic predisposition. Abdominal palpation following a feed is usually diagnostic and reveals an 'olive sized' epigastric mass, the 'pyloric tumour'. Ultrasound is useful to confirm the diagnosis in equivocal cases.

Ultrasound Features
- Pyloric muscle thickness >3 mm.
- Pyloric canal length >16 mm.
- Prominent peristaltic waves fail to allow relaxation of the pylorus and normal gastric emptying.
- Anechoic mass with central echogenic gas – 'bull's eye' sign; it is seen when the pylorus is imaged in a transverse plane.

Hints

This examination is best performed after a small clear feed with the infant turned slightly to the right to optimise the scan window. Long axis measurements are more reproducible than short axis ones.

Pyloric muscle thickness is measured as the distance between the echogenic mucosa and the serosal lining in a longitudinal plane.

Pylorospasm is a close differential diagnosis to consider – the pyloric musculature is of normal thickness with a prominent echogenic mucosa and the pylorus will generally open normally if observation is continued following a feed.

CASE 3

An 8-month-old girl presents with intermittent left upper-quadrant abdominal pain and a palpable mass.

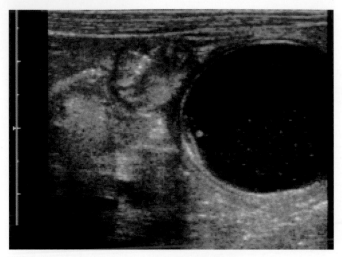

TS epigastrium

Q1. What is the diagnosis?

A1. Duplication cyst

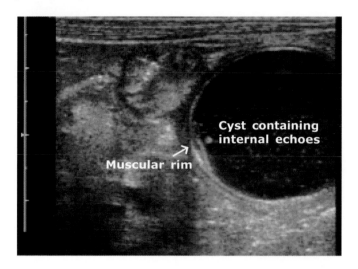

Cyst containing
internal echoes

Muscular rim

Notes

Duplication cysts are enteric mucosal-lined structures located in the mesenteric side of the bowel wall and are caused by an abnormality of gut recanalisation during early foetal life. The majority are small and asymptomatic but large cysts can present with intermittent vomiting due to obstruction of the bowel by the cyst or more acutely following torsion of the adjacent bowel around the cyst. Some may contain ectopic gastric mucosa which can bleed causing abdominal pain.

Ultrasound Features

- Thick-walled cystic mass
- Inner echogenic mucosal lining and outer echo-poor muscle layer– 'muscular rim sign'
- May contain internal echoes (mucus or haemorrhage)

Hints

Differential diagnoses include omental, mesenteric, choledochal cysts, and in girls, ovarian cysts. However, the characteristic 'muscular rim sign' helps distinguish a duplication cyst apart from these entities.

CASE 4

An 8-month-old male infant presents with vomiting, bloody stools and a palpable mass.

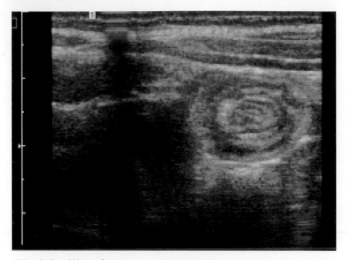

TS right iliac fossa

Q1. What is the diagnosis?

A1. Intussusception

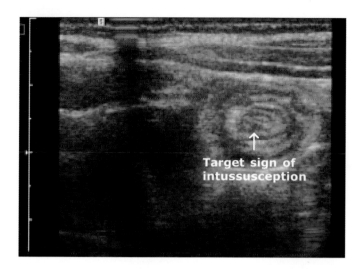

Notes

Intussusception represents telescope-like invagination of a segment of intestinal tract into the lumen of the adjacent intestine. It is a leading cause of bowel obstruction in childhood with most cases occuring in the first 2 years of life. It is thought to be caused by hypertrophied Peyer's patches (small bowel lymphoid tissue), but occasionally, particularly in the older child, a polyp, Meckel's diverticulum or rarely malignancy, e.g., lymphoma, can act as a 'lead point'. Ultrasound readily confirms the diagnosis.

Ultrasound Features
- Alternating hypo- and hyper-echoic layers with central echogenic fat
- Target' sign when viewed in transverse section
- 'Pseudokidney sign' when viewed in longitudinal section

Hints

Intussusception is a surgical emergency as there is a high risk of bowel infarction if left untreated. Radiological techniques such as hydrostatic or pneumatic reduction have a high success rate and are routinely used as the first line of management, unless there are signs of acute peritonitis, where urgent laparotomy is indicated.

CASE 5

A premature infant (28 weeks) undergoes a transcranial ultrasound scan.

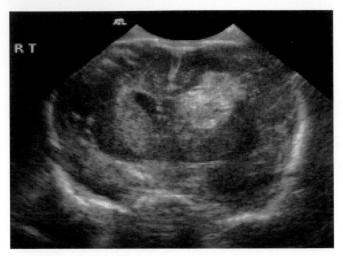

TS lateral ventricles

Q1. What is the diagnosis?

A1. Neonatal intraventricular haemorrhage with parenchymal involvement

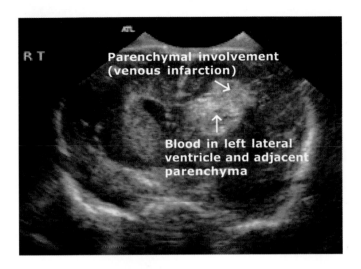

Notes

Intraventricular haemorrhage arises as a result of bleeding in the thin-walled veins of the highly vascular subependymal tissue in the floor of the lateral ventricles. It is a feature of prematurity as beyond 34 weeks the subependymal germinal matrix has largely involuted following the migration of immature neuronal and glial cells to the developing brain. Hypoxia, acidosis, unstable blood pressure and hypercapnia are significant predisposing factors. In severe cases ventricular distension results in venous congestion and subsequent venous infarction in the adjacent peri-ventricular white matter.

Ultrasound Features

- Variable depending on size, age and severity of bleed. The haemorrhage is initially highly echogenic and gradually becomes less echogenic as it resolves.
- The mildest degree of haemorrhage is confined to the subependymal germinal matrix. Larger haemorrhages result in intraventricular bleeding and ventricular dilatation. Secondary adjacent parenchymal involvement due to venous infarction may be seen in the most severe cases.
- Post haemorrhagic hydrocephalus is an important complication following intraventricular haemorrhage and is related to the size of the initial bleed.

CASE 6

A two-week-old female is brought to the paediatrician after her mother discovered a mass in the left flank.

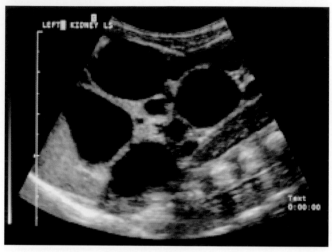

LS left flank

Q1. What is the diagnosis?

A1. Multicystic dysplastic kidney

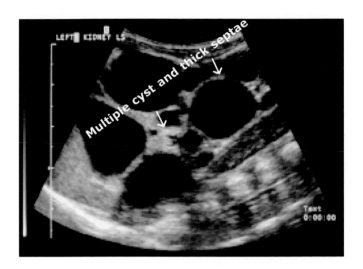

Notes
Multicystic dysplastic kidney (MCDK) is a developmental anomaly of the urinary tract, where the presence of ureteric atresia results in the failure of normal renal parenchymal development. It is unilateral in the majority and fatal if bilateral. MCDK is the second commonest cause of a palpable abdominal mass in neonates (congenital hydronephrosis is more common). MCDK is distinguished from severe hydronephrosis by the lack of communication between the cysts, absence of normal intervening renal tissue and complete absence of function on DMSA scan.

Ultrasound Features
- Multiple non-communicating cysts with thick septa.
- Absence of normal renal parenchyma and sinus fat.
- Multiple small echogenic foci of primitive mesenchyme may be visualised between multiple cysts.

Hints
30% of patients have associated anomalies of the contralateral kidney such as vesicoureteric reflux.

CASE 7

A 4-year-old child presents with a large right-sided abdominal mass.

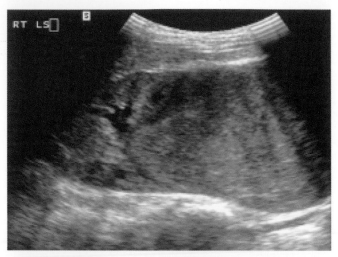

LS right kidney

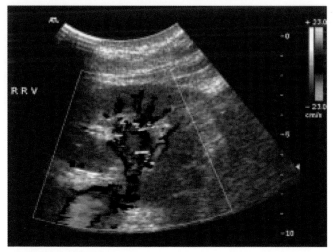

LS right kidney

Q1. What is the diagnosis?
Q2. Why is the renal vein being assessed?

A1. Wilms tumour
A2. To assess for venous invasion

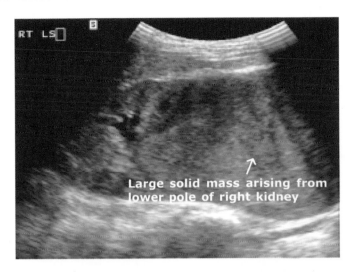

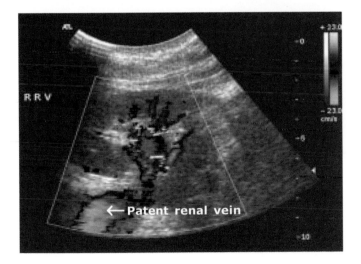

Notes

Wilms tumour is the most common malignant neoplasm of childhood. It arises from undifferentiated nephrogenic rests and is associated with hemihypertrophy, Beckwith-Weidemann and DRASH syndromes. These tumours are often large (>10 cm) and the role of imaging is to identify site of origin of the mass, assess local spread and vascular invasion.

Ultrasound Features
- Large mixed echogenicity intrarenal mass
- Contralateral kidney involved in 10%
- Calcification seen in 10%

Hints
Neuroblastoma, in contrast to Wilms tumour, is calcified in 90% of cases, usually crosses the midline and encases vessels rather than displacing them.

Wilms tumours have a propensity to spread via venous invasion and Doppler interrogation of the renal vein and IVC is essential.

CASE 8

A 6-week-old girl presents with jaundice. Pale stools, and blood tests reveal a conjugated hyperbilirubinemia.

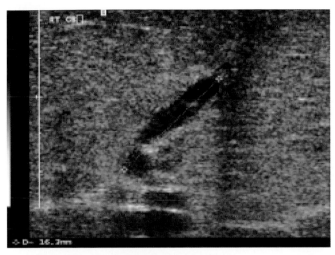

Porta hepatis (high-frequency probe)

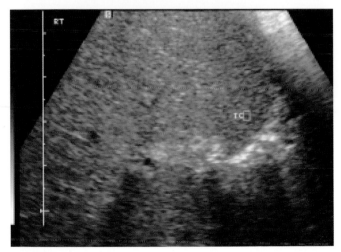

Porta hepatis (high-frequency probe)

Q1. What are the relevant findings?
Q2. What is the diagnosis?

A1. Small gallbladder, triangular cord sign (image 2)
A2. Biliary atresia

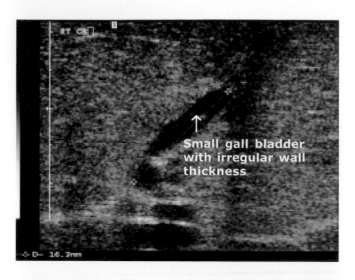

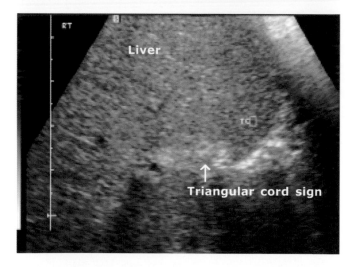

Notes

Biliary atresia is a rare but serious condition. Imaging is important to distinguish it from idiopathic neonatal hepatitis as both present with conjugate hyperbilirubinaemia in the first month of life. Neonatal hepatitis is a non-surgical disease, whereas biliary atresia requires operative intervention via a portoenterostomy (Kasai procedure) with best results achieved within the first 8 weeks of life.

Ultrasound Features
- Echogenic structure at the porta hepatis – 'triangular cord sign'.
- Abnormal gallbladder or non-visualisation of the gallbladder in the fasted patient.
- Gallbladder may be small, have irregular wall, abnormal shape (examine with high-frequency probe).
- Common bile duct is usually absent.

Hints
The 'triangular cord sign' represents the fibrotic remnant of the extra hepatic biliary tree and when present is highly specific for biliary atresia. Using a combination of ultrasound features can increase the accuracy of diagnosis.

Excretion of isotope into the small bowel demonstrated by hepatobiliary scintigraphy (IDA scan) excludes biliary atresia; however, non-excretion can occur in both biliary atresia and neonatal hepatitis.

CASE 9

A 3-year-old child presents to A & E with a limp and complains of a painful left hip.

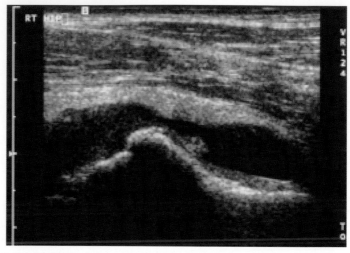

LS left hip

Q1. What is the differential diagnosis?

A1. Septic arthritis, haemorrhagic effusion, juvenile rheumatoid arthritis

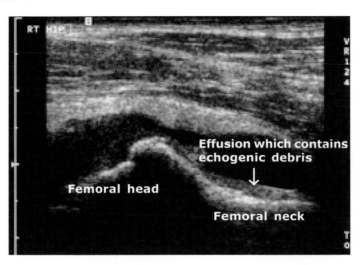

Notes
The key differential diagnoses for a child with hip pain and effusion are septic arthritis and transient synovitis (irritable hip). Septic arthritis is an orthopaedic emergency requiring urgent joint washout, whereas transient synovitis is a benign self-limiting condition. Ultrasound is used to confirm the presence of joint fluid and to guide diagnostic aspiration where appropriate.

Ultrasound Features
- Echo-poor fluid collection distending the joint capsule.
- Echogenic debris in the fluid may be seen in cases of infection, haemorrhage or with inflammatory effusions in cases of juvenile arthritis.

Hints
Ultrasound has high accuracy for detection of a hip effusion, but cannot reliably tell septic arthritis from transient synovitis. Clinical and biochemical correlation are always essential.

CASE 10

A 15-year-old boy with epilepsy and learning difficulties is referred for renal ultrasound.

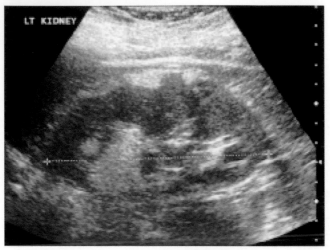

LS left kidney

Q1. What is the diagnosis?
Q2. What hereditary disorder does he have?

A1. Multiple angiomyolipomas
A2. Tuberous sclerosis

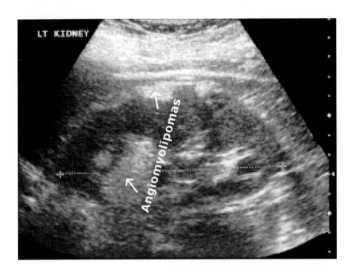

Notes
Tuberous sclerosis is an autosomal dominant condition which affects multiple organ systems including the CNS, skin and kidneys. Renal lesions occur in 50% of patients and comprise multiple cysts, multiple angiomyolipomas and renal cell carcinomas. Angiomyolipomas are benign mixed tumours composed of blood vessels, muscle and fat. When found in children/young adults they are invariably associated with tuberous sclerosis.

Ultrasound Features
- Cortical-based, well-defined, echo-bright masses.
- One-third cast a post-acoustic shadow.

Hints
Most angiomyolipomas are small (<2 cm), occur sporadically and are asymptomatic.

Large lesions (>4 cm) are usually associated with tuberous sclerosis and carry a significant risk of spontaneous retroperitoneal haemorrhage. Vascular embolisation may be considered to prevent potentially life-threatening complications.

CASE 11

An 8-year-old boy under investigation for recurrent urinary tract infections is admitted with high fever and malaise.

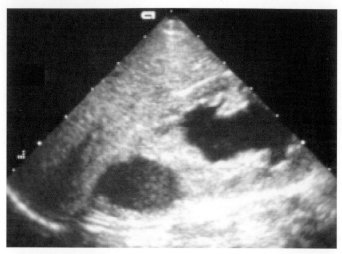

LS right kidney

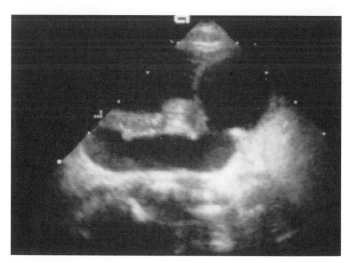

LS bladder

Q1. What is the diagnosis?
Q2. What complication has occurred?

A1. Duplex kidney
A2. Obstructed, infected system

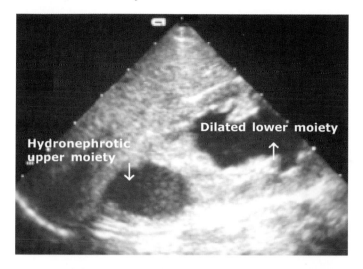

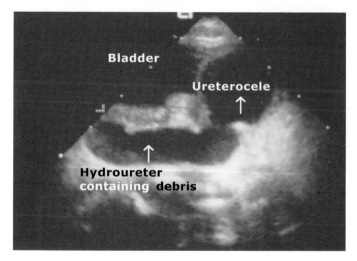

Notes

A duplex kidney is when the renal collecting system is divided by a bridge of parenchymal tissue with each moiety being drained by separate ureters. The ureter draining the upper-moiety usually inserts into the bladder inferior and medial to the lower-moiety ureter (Weigert-Meyer rule). In some duplex kidneys the ureters fuse prior to entry into the bladder.

Ultrasound Features
- Parenchymal bridge can be difficult to see.
- Upper-moiety ureter is often associated with a ureterocele.
- Lower-moiety ureter is associated with vesicoureteric reflux.

Hints
Suspect a duplex system when a fluid collection is seen at the upper pole of a kidney.

The upper moiety is usually non-functioning on isotope scans.

The obstructed ureter/upper moiety is prone to secondary infection (pyonephrosis).

CASE 12

A 12-year-old boy presents with a 6-hour history of left groin and testicular pain.

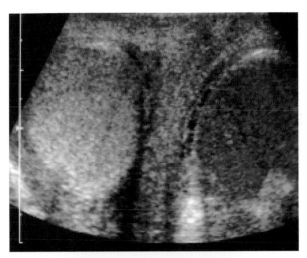

TS both testes

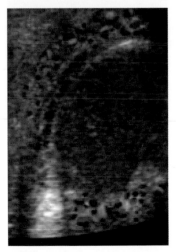

TS left testis with colour Doppler

Q1. What is the diagnosis?

A1. Left testicular torsion

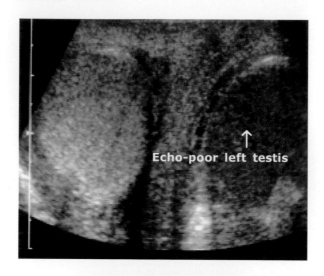

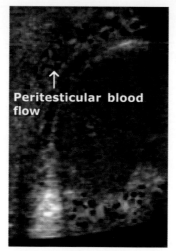

Notes

Testicular torsion is a surgical emergency caused by twisting of the spermatic cord. Venous return is initially obstructed which raises intra-testicular pressure leading to arterial compromise and infarction if not urgently relieved. Surgical exploration should not be delayed if there is a strong clinical suspicion, but imaging is useful in equivocal cases. The majority of testes can be salvaged if operated on within 6 hours.

Ultrasound Features
Grey scale imaging
- < 6 h Normal echogenicity
- 6–12 h Diffusely echo-poor
- >12 h Heterogeneous echotexture

Colour Doppler imaging
- Reduced/absent intra-testicular blood flow is the hallmark.
- Peri-testicular blood flow is normal or increased.
- Twisting of spermatic cord vessels: 'whirlpool sign'.

Hints
Doppler ultrasound has a sensitivity and specificity of >95%.

False negatives
Can occur in the first few hours when only venous flow is occluded and also in cases of intermittent torsion/ detorsion.

False positives
Can occur with incorrect machine set up, especially when imaging the prepubescent testis in which flow can be difficult to detect normally.

CASE 13

A 15-year-old boy presents with bloody diarrhoea and severe abdominal pain.

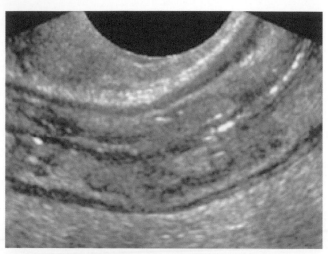

LS right iliac fossa

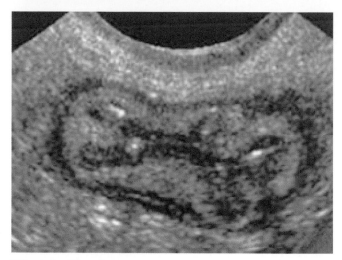

TS right iliac fossa

Q1. What is the diagnosis?

A1. Crohn's disease

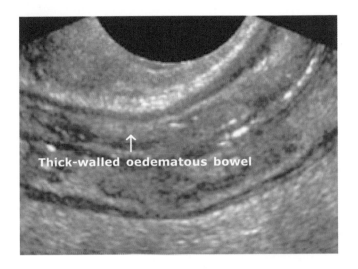

Notes

Crohn's disease is a chronic granulomatous inflammatory disorder of the gastrointestinal tract with a tendency towards remission and relapse. It can affect anywhere from mouth to anus often involving multiple discontinuous sites. The terminal ileum and ascending colon are involved in 80% of cases. The disease may begin at any age, but onset most commonly occurs between 15 and 30 years of age. Most patients present with recurrent episodes of diarrhoea frequently associated with weight loss, abdominal pain and low-grade fever.

Ultrasound Features
- Bowel wall thickening (>3 mm)
- Mural hyperaemia with colour Doppler
- Fibrofatty proliferation adjacent to involved segments
- Low-volume mesenteric lymphadenopathy

Hints

Look for complications of Crohn's disease which in children include abscess formation and intestinal obstruction.

In acute-on-chronic presentations the presence of a fistula or perforation should also be considered. MRI or CT may be useful adjuncts in such cases when complications are not readily apparent on ultrasound.

CASE 14

A 5-year-old boy presents with high-grade fever 2 weeks following a chest infection.

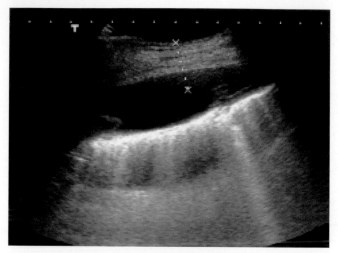

Transverse image along chest wall

Q1. What is the diagnosis?

A1. Empyema

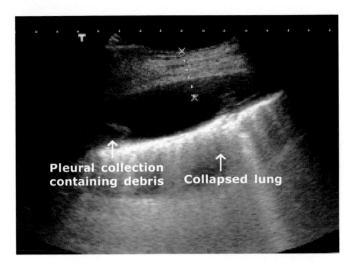

Notes
Empyema is a purulent collection within the pleural cavity which most commonly results from transformation of a parapneumonic effusion. Patients describe pleuritic chest pain and are systemically unwell. Initial treatment is with antibiotics and chest tube drainage, but this may be unsuccessful, especially with multiloculated collections. Surgical techniques such as video-assisted thorascopic debridement or thoracotomy and decortication may ultimately be required.

Ultrasound Features
- Echo-poor collection in the pleural space
- Contains internal septations or solid components

Hints
Ultrasound is a safe and effective means of guiding chest tube placement. The Seldinger technique is preferably used whereby the pleural space is first entered with an introducer needle through which a guidewire is advanced. Dilators are then used to open up a tract, the drain is 'rail-roaded' over the guidewire and the guidewire is finally withdrawn.

Chapter 6

Cardiovascular

CASE 1

A 65-year-old woman is referred with a groin mass 24 hours after coronary angioplasty.

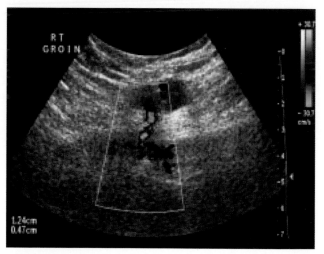

LS right groin

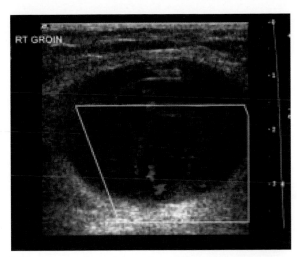

LS right groin with colour Doppler (zoom)

Q1. What is the diagnosis?
Q2. What radiological treatment may be offered?

A1. Femoral artery pseudo-aneurysm
A2. Ultrasound-guided thrombin injection

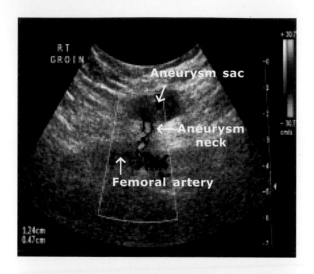

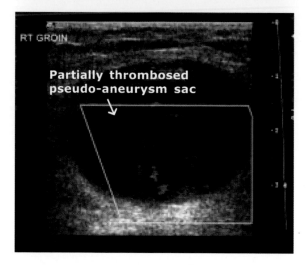

Notes

A pseudo-aneurysm (or 'false' aneurysm) is caused by a focal disruption of the arterial wall. The resultant high-pressure leak is contained by adjacent tissues and haematoma. Pseudo-aneurysms occur in <1% of diagnostic angiograms and in around 3–5% of interventional procedures; the larger the catheter used the higher the risk.

Ultrasound Features

- Echo-poor 'sac' seen adjacent to the femoral artery.
- The 'sac' may contain internal echoes (partial thrombosis).
- 'Swirling' blood flow seen within the 'sac' using colour Doppler.
- A communicating 'neck' links the parent artery to the 'sac'.
- Bi-directional flow pattern is seen within the neck using spectral Doppler

Hints

The main differential diagnosis is a groin haematoma with transmitted pulsation from the adjacent artery. A haematoma has no neck, does not display internal blood flow.

Ultrasound-guided compression or thrombin injection can be used to treat thin-necked aneurysms.

CASE 2

A 50-year-old woman has a swollen tender right leg one week following hip replacement surgery.

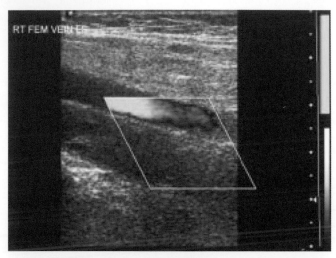

LS right SFV with power Doppler

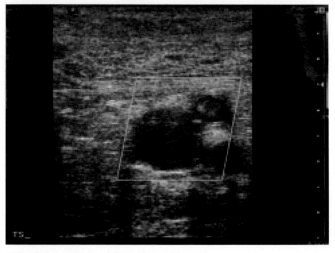

TS right SFV with colour Doppler

Q1. What is the diagnosis?
Q2. What complication can occur with this condition?

A1. Femoral vein deep venous thrombosis (DVT)
A2. Pulmonary embolism

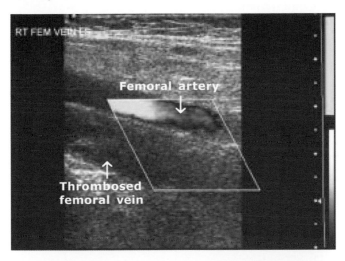

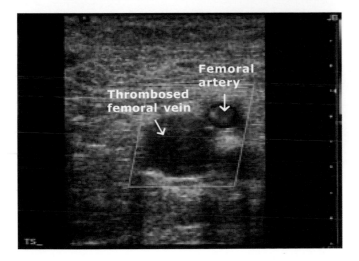

Notes

DVT usually presents as a painful swollen limb. Risk factors include pregnancy, intravenous drug use, immobility and hyper-coagulable states. The left leg is more commonly affected than the right which is thought to be due to compressive effects on the left iliac vein by the crossing right iliac artery. Untreated there is a high risk of pulmonary embolism.

Ultrasound Features

Acute
- Dilated vein containing echo-poor thrombus.
- Non-compressible and absent colour flow.

Chronic
- Echo-bright thrombus in a contracted vein.
- Colour flow may be seen within it due to partial re-canalisation.

Hints

If a thrombus is detected its degree of proximal extension should be assessed.

Up to 25% of people have duplicated femoral and/or popliteal veins.

In the early stages, thrombus may be non-occlusive and the vein will therefore be partially compressible.

If a scan is negative for DVT, check for conditions which can mimic it:
- Intramuscular haematoma
- Ruptured Baker's cyst
- Cellulitis (oedematous subcutaneous tissues)

CASE 3

A 50-year-old woman with rheumatoid arthritis is referred with an acute swollen and painful right calf, query DVT?

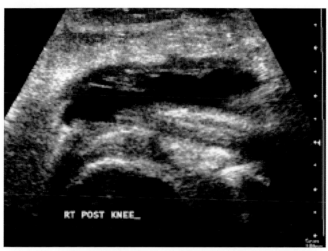

TS right popliteal fossa

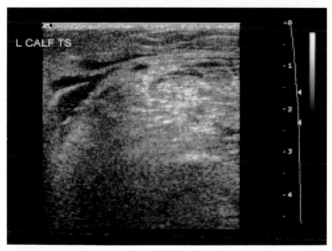

TS right mid calf

Q1. What is the diagnosis?
Q2. What complication has occurred?

A1. Baker's cyst
A2. Rupture into the calf tissues

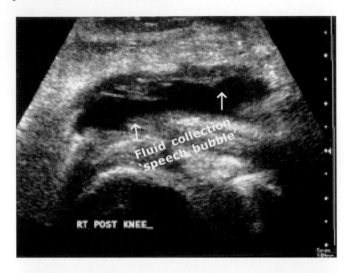

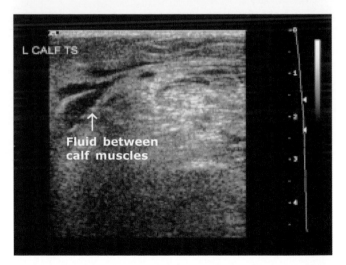

Notes

A Baker's cyst is a synovial fluid–filled outpouching from the posterior joint capsule of the knee. It is most commonly located on the medial side of the popliteal fossa between the medial head of gastrocnemius and semimembranosus tendon. There is an association with rheumatoid arthritis and meniscal injuries.

Ultrasound Features
- Oval/crescent-shaped echo-free collection
- Communicates with the knee joint – 'speech bubble sign'

Hints
If a Baker's cyst ruptures, the synovial fluid tracks down into the calf and can mimic a DVT clinically. Look for fluid collections in the subcutaneous tissues and between the posterior calf muscles.

CASE 4

A 40-year-old man presents with pain and 'lumps' in his left calf.

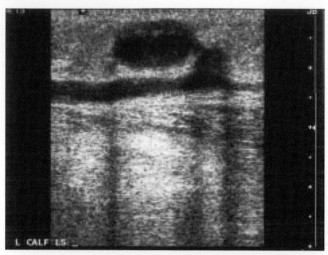

LS left calf

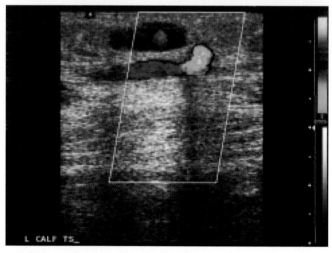

LS left calf with colour Doppler

Q1. What is the diagnosis?

A1. Varicose veins

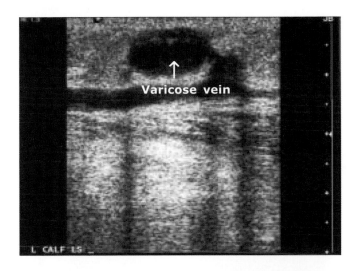

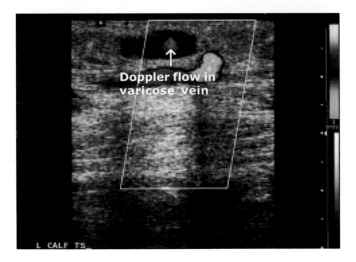

Notes

Varicose veins are caused by incompetent vein valves which allow reflux of blood from the deep into the superficial venous system. The thin-walled superficial veins dilate under the increased pressure. The majority are idiopathic (primary). Secondary causes include a prior DVT which has rendered the vein valves incompetent.

Ultrasound Features
- Dilated tortuous superficial veins
- Display colour Doppler flow

Hints
A common complication of varicose veins is inflammation (thrombophlebitis). The varicosities appear thick walled with surrounding soft tissue oedema.

CASE 5

A 60-year-old man is referred for carotid Doppler examination with recurrent episodes of syncope and ataxia.

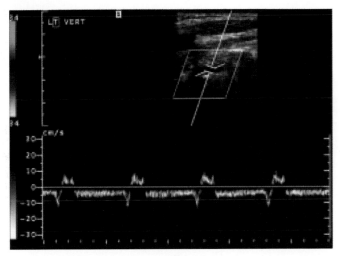

Spectral Doppler left vertebral artery

Q1. What is the diagnosis?

A1. Left subclavian steal syndrome

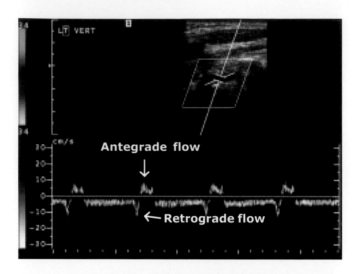

Notes

Subclavian steal is caused by narrowing (partial steal) or occlusion (complete steal) of the proximal subclavian (or brachiocephalic) artery. Blood flows in a retrograde direction down the ipsilateral vertebral artery to supply the distal subclavian – diverting flow away from the vertebrobasilar circulation. This can cause syncopal episodes, vertigo and ataxia, classically induced by exercising the arm on the affected side.

Ultrasound Features

Partial Steal

- Antegrade flow in vertebral artery during diastole.
- Retrograde flow in vertebral artery during systole.
- Exercising arm on the affected side exaggerates the wave for change.
- Brachial artery on affected side has a monophasic waveform.

Complete Steal

- Retrograde flow throughout the cardiac cycle.

Hints

The normal vertebral artery Doppler waveform is low resistance with forward (antegrade) flow throughout the cardiac cycle.

The normal brachial artery waveform is tri-phasic.

Asking the patient to exercise their arm while scanning the vertebral artery will exaggerate the waveform change.

CASE 6

A 40-year-old woman presents with a 3-month history of increasing breathlessness and reduced exercise capacity. A pansystolic murmur can be heard on auscultation.

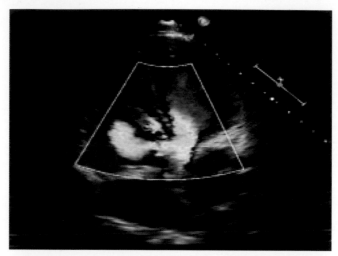

4-chamber view of the heart with colour Doppler

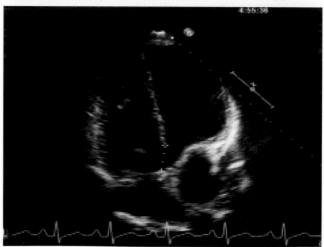

4-chamber view of the heart

Q1. What is the diagnosis?

A1. Ventricular septal defect causing pulmonary hypertension

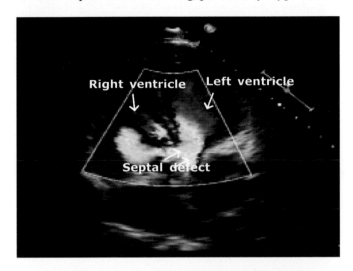

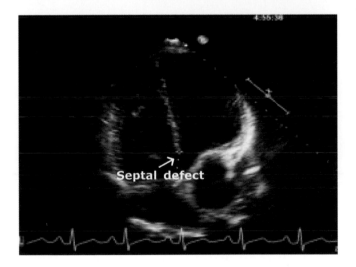

Notes

Ventricular septal defect (VSD) is the most common congenital cardiac defect. Associated anomalies include aortic coarctation, patent ductus arteriosus, tetralogy of Fallot and trisomy 21. Pressure differences between the low-resistance right ventricle and the high-resistance left ventricle create a left-to-right shunt. The increased load on the right heart leads to pulmonary hypertension and right heart failure. If left untreated, pulmonary resistance can rise above systemic leading to shunt reversal and cyanosis (Eisenmenger's syndrome).

Ultrasound Features
- Perimembranous defects account for the majority.
- Echo 'dropout' adjacent to the defect.
- Colour Doppler displays the shunt.

Hints
A third of small VSDs close spontaneously in early childhood. Larger shunts require corrective surgery or trans-catheterisation closure.

CASE 7

A 70-year-old man under investigation for a recent TIA is referred for carotid Doppler examination.

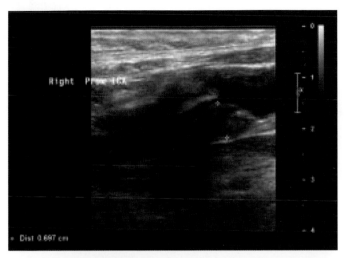

LS right carotid bulb

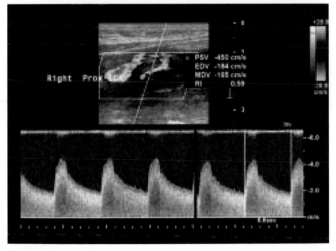

Spectral Doppler right ICA

Q1. What is seen in image 1?
Q2. What is the diagnosis?

A1. Large plaque at the ICA origin
A2. ICA stenosis >70%

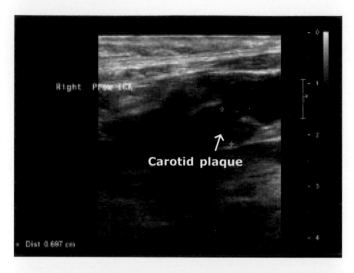

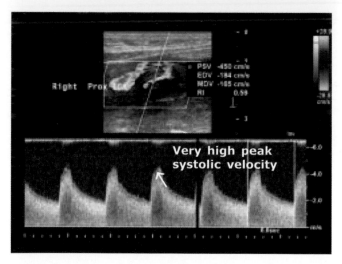

Notes
Imaging of the extracranial carotid vessels is routinely performed following a stroke or TIA to assess for significant luminal narrowing by atherosclerotic plaques. Ultrasound and other non-invasive imaging techniques like MRI have largely replaced the need for invasive catheter angiography. ICA stenosis between 70 and 99% has been shown to benefit from endarterectomy surgery.

Ultrasound Features (>70% stenosis)
- Peak systolic velocity in the ICA >230 cm/sec
- ICA/CCA peak systolic velocity gradient >4

Supportive Features
- Spectral broadening of ICA waveform – 'filling in' under curve
- ECA waveform shows increased diastolic flow – 'ICA like'

Hints
Features of the normal ECA waveform
- Arises antero-medial to the ICA and has side branches in the neck
- Demonstrates the 'temporal tapping' phenomena
- Waveform has a characteristic notch and may dip below the baseline

Features of the normal ICA waveform
- No side branches in the neck
- No 'temporal tapping' phenomena
- Has a low-resistance waveform, i.e., high end-diastolic flow

Limitations of ultrasound
- Calcified plaques can interfere with Doppler interrogation.
- Inability to visualise ICA lesions near the skull base.
- Inability to image the origins of the neck vessels.

CASE 8

A 60-year-old man with weight loss is referred for a routine abdominal ultrasound.

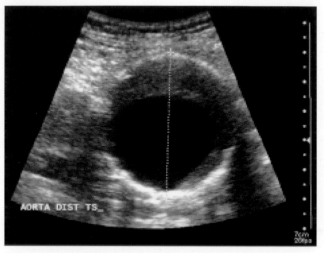

TS aorta

Q1. What is the diagnosis?
Q2. What action should be taken?

A1. Abdominal aortic aneurysm
A2. Contact the vascular surgeons

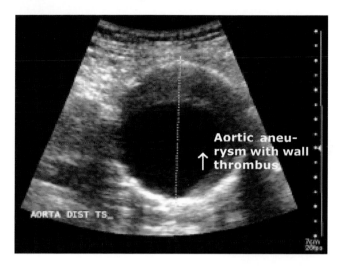

Notes
Abdominal aortic aneurysms (AAA) are defined as focal areas of aortic dilatation that exceed 3 cm in maximal diameter. Most AAAs result from atherosclerosis, they are more common in men and most originate below the level of the renal arteries. Over time AAAs enlarge and surgical or endovascular repair is considered when they exceed 5 cm because of a greatly increased risk of rupture.

Ultrasound Features
• Localised dilation of abdominal aorta >3 cm
• Filling defects with colour Doppler (mural thrombus)

Hints
The following features are associated with a high risk of rupture:
• Size >6 cm
• Growth by >5 mm in 6 months
• Abdominal/back pain

Any of these features should prompt discussion with the vascular surgeons.

Always assess if the origin of the aneurysm is above or below the renal arteries as this has implications regarding surgical technique. This can be difficult due to bowel gas shadowing and aneurysmal distortion of anatomy; one clue is to find the SMA origin in longitudinal section – the renal vessels arise about 1cm below this.

CASE 9

A 65-year-old man with multiple myeloma is referred for ultrasound venogram because of an acutely swollen right calf. Examination of the popliteal and above-knee veins shows these vessels to be patent.

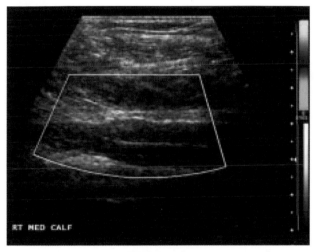

LS right posterior tibial veins

Q1. What is the diagnosis?

A1. Calf DVT

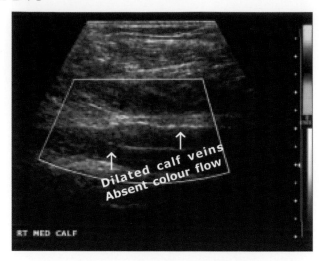

Notes

Below-knee DVT is more difficult to diagnose than popliteal or femoral vein thrombosis because of the small calibre of the vessels. Treatment of isolated below-knee DVT remains controversial. The safety of withholding therapy has been demonstrated, but around 20% will subsequently propagate into the popliteal veins with the potential to embolise. If treatment is withheld serial scans are required to assess for proximal extension.

Ultrasound Features
- Dilated deep calf veins containing echo-poor thrombus
- Absence of colour flow

Hints

Locate the posterior tibial veins by placing the probe along the medial calf and angle slightly laterally. These paired veins run alongside the posterior tibial artery deep to the tibia.

Locate the anterior tibial veins by scanning along the lateral calf and angle slightly medially. These veins run between the tibia and fibula above the interosseous membrane.

Absence of colour flow should not be used on its own to make the diagnosis as normal calf veins often have undetectable flow. Squeezing the ankle while scanning makes blood flow easier to detect.

CASE 10

A 50-year-old man presents with a swollen right thigh. Clinically there is tenderness over the medial aspect. He is referred for an ultrasound venogram, query DVT.

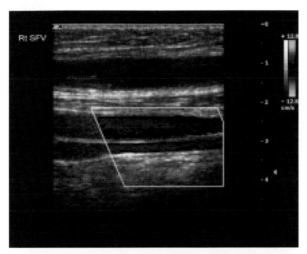

LS right thigh with colour Doppler

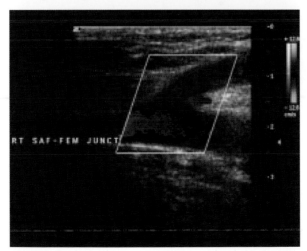

LS sapheno-femoral junction with colour Doppler

Q1. What is the diagnosis?
Q2. What is a recognised complication?

A1. Thrombophlebitis of the long saphenous vein
A2. Clot propagation into deep venous system and pulmonary embolism

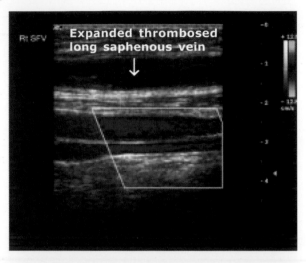

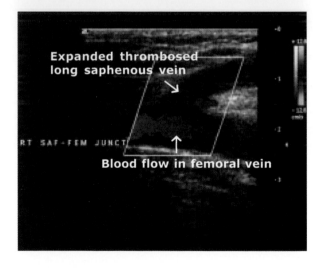

Notes
Thrombosis of this superficial vein is associated with hypercoagulable states, smoking and trauma. Patients present with redness, swelling and extreme tenderness over the medial thigh.

Ultrasound Features
- Dilated long saphenous containing echo-poor thrombus
- Absent colour flow in the vein
- Thickened vein wall (phlebitis)

Hints
The long saphenous vein lies just beneath the skin and runs along the medial aspect of the thigh. It terminates by piercing the deep fascia in the region of the groin crease to drain into the femoral vein.

The short saphenous runs along the lateral aspect of the calf and terminates by piercing the deep fascia to join the popliteal vein behind the knee.

The major risk with greater or lesser saphenous vein thrombosis is clot propagation into the deep venous system (up to 50% of cases). This carries a significant risk of pulmonary embolism. Treatment involves anticoagulation or surgical ligation of the sapheno-femoral/ popliteal junction.

CASE 11

A 35-year-old woman who is 3-days post-partum develops sudden onset chest pain and breathlessness. An urgent bedside echocardiogram is performed.

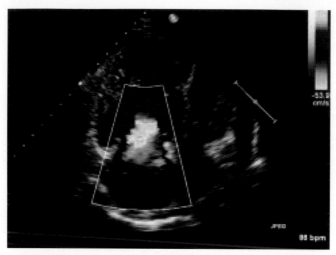

4-chamber view of the heart

Q1. What does this appearance mean?
Q2. What is the most likely diagnosis?

A1. Severe right heart strain

A2. Acute pulmonary embolism (PE)

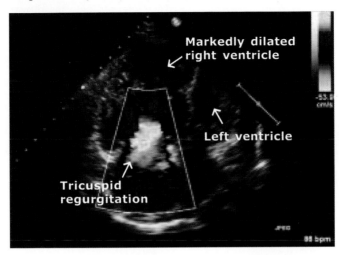

Notes
More than 90% of PEs arise from venous thrombosis within the deep leg or pelvic veins. Pressure effects by the gravid uterus in combination with increased blood viscosity predispose to PE during pregnancy. Entrapment of emboli within the pulmonary arterial tree causes cessation of distal blood flow and an increase in pulmonary vascular resistance. Large or multiple emboli can cause death secondary to severe right ventricular strain and circulatory collapse. Echocardiography facilitates bedside assessment of right ventricular strain in a haemodynamically unstable patient.

Ultrasound Features
- Dilated right heart chambers (right ventricle larger than left)
- Tricuspid regurgitation

Hints
The presence of hypotension (shock) defines a threefold to sevenfold increase in mortality, with the majority of deaths occurring within one hour of presentation. Signs of right heart strain correlate with a worse clinical outcome and may prompt treatment with thrombolysis or catheter embolectomy.

CASE 12

A 45-year-old woman with a history of metastatic breast cancer presents with increasing breathlessness.

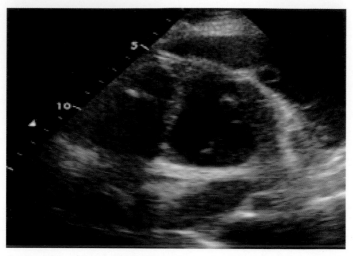

4-chamber view of the heart

A1. Pericardial effusion

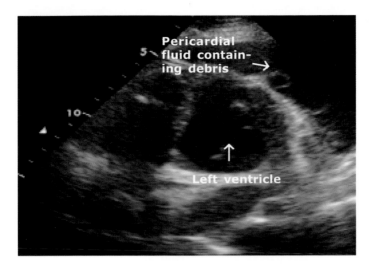

Notes

Pericardial effusion is caused by obstruction of venous or lymphatic drainage from the heart. Common causes include heart failure, renal insufficiency, infection and neoplasia (particularly metastatic disease from lung and breast carcinoma). Echocardiography is considered the primary imaging modality for initial evaluation.

Ultrasound Features

- Echo-poor pericardial collection
- May contain internal echoes or solid components depending upon the aetiology

Hints

Excessive accumulation of pericardial fluid can cause cardiac tamponade. This is a life-threatening condition that results from heart compression secondary to accumulation of fluid or tissue within the pericardial cavity. Intrapericardial pressure becomes sufficiently raised so as to compress the heart with resultant haemodynamic impairment. This leads to limited cardiac inflow, decreased stroke volume, and reduced blood pressure (cardiogenic shock). The thin right-sided chambers are the first to be compressed in the setting of tamponade and right atrial collapse, which occurs in late diastole or early systole, is one of the earliest echocardiographic signs. Treatment of tamponade is by needle pericardiocentesis which can be performed using echocardiographic, fluoroscopic, or CT guidance.

Chapter 7

Testicular

CASE 1

A 75-year-old man who suffers from recurrent UTIs is referred because of a swollen tender right testicle.

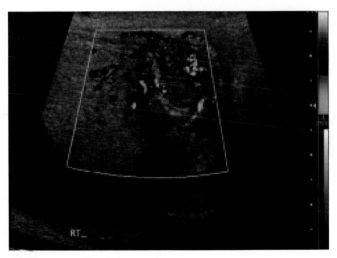

TS lower pole right testis

Q1. What is the diagnosis?

A1. Epididymitis

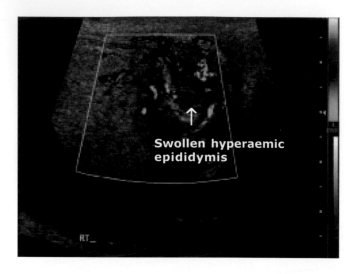

Notes
Epididymitis is caused by ascending spread of infection, most commonly urinary pathogens, e.g., *E.coli* in the elderly or sexually transmitted infections, e.g., *Chlamydia*, in young males

Ultrasound Features
- Swollen (>3 mm) echo-poor epididymis; tail is most common part affected.
- Colour Doppler flow is increased over affected area in the acute phase.
- There will often be a reactive hydrocele.
- Oedematous thickening of the scrotal skin may also be seen.

Hints
If longstanding or untreated, an abscess may develop (echo-poor collection of pus with internal echo-bright debris).

Occasionally infection can spread to involve the testis (orchitis). Look carefully for any signs of this (swollen testis containing echo-poor areas).

CASE 2

A 19-year-old man is referred by his GP after feeling a 'lump' in his right testis.

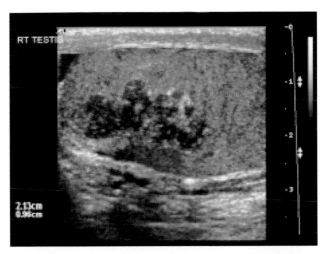

LS right testis

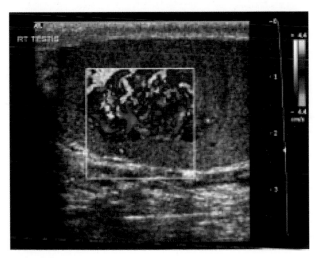

LS right testis with colour Doppler

Q1. What is the diagnosis?

A1. Testicular tumour

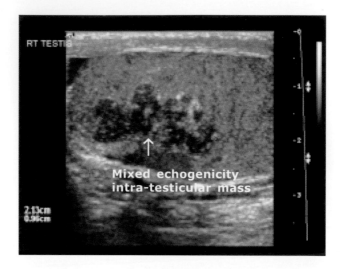

Notes
Testicular tumours are the commonest neoplasm in young men. Risk factors include cryptorchidism (undescended testis), microlithiasis and a positive family history. The majority are of germ cell origin with seminoma being the commonest histological subtype. Serum tumour marker levels are elevated in 80% of cases at time of diagnosis.

Ultrasound Features
- Intra-testicular mass lesion.
- Can be echo-poor, cystic or of mixed echogenicity.
- Some tumour types may contain coarse calcifications.
- Intra-lesional blood flow.

Hints
As a rule most intra-testicular mass lesions are malignant.

An abdominal ultrasound should also be performed to assess for tumour spread, e.g., para-aortic lymphadenopathy. A chest X-ray should be requested to assess for lung metastases and a urologist contacted to arrange urgent clinical assessment.

Patients who have previously had a testicular tumour require regular surveillance scans of the other testis as there is a 5–10% chance of a contralateral tumour developing.

CASE 3

A 40-year-old man is being investigated for subfertility.

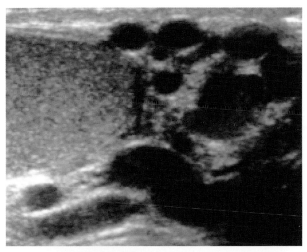

Lower pole right testis

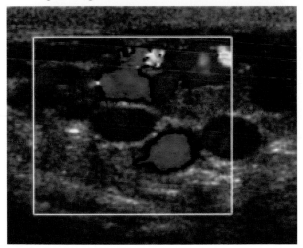

Lower pole right testis with colour Doppler

Q1. What is the diagnosis?
Q2. What should be scanned next?

A1. Varicocele
A2. Kidneys

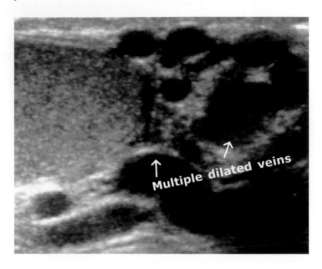

Notes
Varicoceles are dilations of the pampiniform veins that drain the testis, and are caused by incompetent vein valves. They are common (around 10% of males), with 90% occurring on the left side. Clinically they may cause a dull scrotal ache and soft scrotal swelling.

Ultrasound Features
- Tortuous dilated (>2 mm) tubular structures
- Located posterior to the epididymis
- Increase in size on straining or standing upright
- Display strong colour or power Doppler flow

Hints
A renal scan should be performed as varicoceles can occasionally be caused by a renal tumour invading the renal vein and obstructing venous return from the testicular veins.

Varicoceles are associated with subfertility and can be effectively treated by coil embolisation.

CASE 4

A 44-year-old man is referred with persistent dull scrotal ache that has been present since his vasectomy 3 months previously.

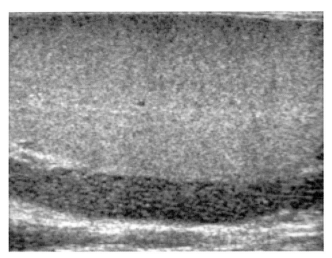

LS right testis

Q1. What is the diagnosis?

A1. Post-vasectomy changes

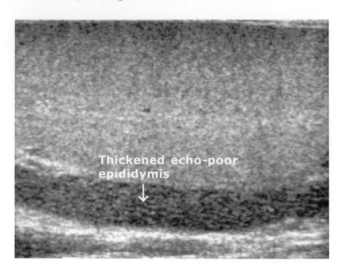

Notes

Up to 20% of post-vasectomy patients complain of chronic discomfort for months/years following the procedure. This is thought to be caused by a combination of back pressure effects and low-grade inflammatory reaction.

Ultrasound Features
- Epididymis is thickened (>3 mm) and echo-poor.
- It contains multiple small punctate cystic areas.

Hints

Look carefully for a sperm granuloma caused by sperm extravasation into the epididymis at time of operation. This is a small well-defined echobright epididymal mass which is a common cause of post-vasectomy pain. Spermatoceles are also sometimes seen post vasectomy. These are benign cystic accumulations of sperm, most commonly in the epididymal head. They look like epididymal cysts, but with internal echoes.

CASE 5

A 35-year-old man is referred for testicular ultrasound during investigation for subfertility.

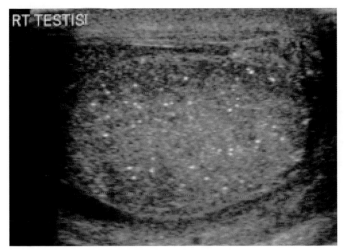

LS right testis

Q1. What is the diagnosis?

A1. Testicular microlithiasis

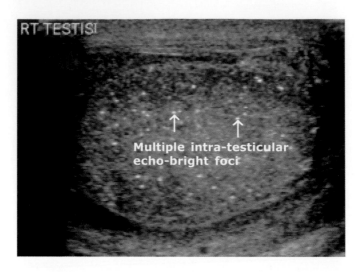

Notes

Microlithiasis is the presence of multiple small calcified foci within the testis. It is usually an incidental finding, but some studies have shown an increased risk of developing a testicular malignancy. They are also associated with subfertility.

Ultrasound Features
- 5 echo-bright foci (each <3 mm) within the body of the testis

Hints

Microlithiasis should not be confused with larger foci of calcification which are usually the result of prior trauma or infection.

Look very carefully for a co-existant testicular tumour (in up to 20% of cases).

These patients should have follow-up scans to monitor for malignancy and perform regular self-examinations.

CASE 6

A 25-year-old man presents with a swollen painful left testis 5 days following a rugby injury.

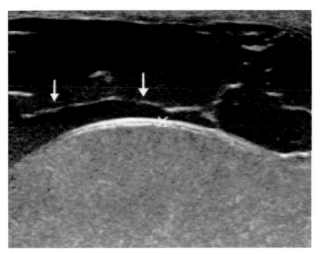

LS left testis

Q1. What is the diagnosis?

A1. Haematocele

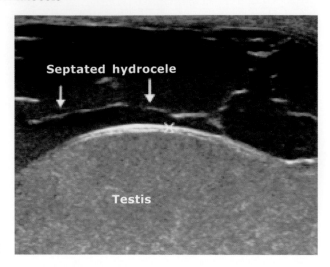

Notes

A hydrocele is fluid accumulation between the two layers of the tunica vaginalis. It can be congenital or acquired.

Congenital – caused by non-closure of the processus vaginalis

Acquired – caused by trauma (haematocele), tumour, inflammation

Ultrasound Features

- Echo-free area typically located on the anterolateral aspect of the testis.
- Fine septations or debris may be seen within the fluid, especially the acquired types (as in this case).

Hints

Ultrasound should also be used to look for injury to the testis, e.g., intratesticular haematoma or testicular disruption (seen as discontinuity of the cortex).

CASE 7

A 42-year-old man is referred for testicular ultrasound having discovered a 'lump' in his right testicle.

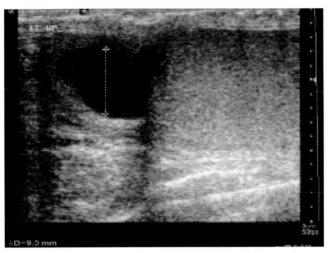

LS left testis upper pole region

Q1. What is the diagnosis?

A1. Epididymal cyst

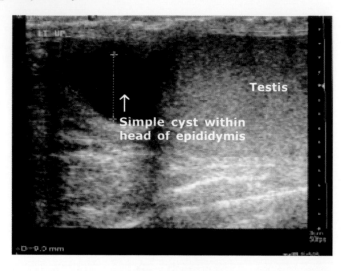

Notes

Epididymal cysts are a common finding (up to 40% of men) and are caused by outpouchings of the epididymal tubules. Such cysts are usually asymptomatic, but if large may present clinically as a smooth firm lump above the testis.

Ultrasound Features

- Most commonly located in the epididymal head
- Displays the features of a simple cyst:
  - Smooth edge
  - Thin wall
  - Echo-free contents
  - Post-acoustic enhancement

Hints

Benign cystic lesions are common findings with testicular ultrasound. They may be intra-testicular, epididymal (as in this case) or para-testicular, e.g., tunica vaginalis cyst. The extratesticular cysts commonly present as 'lumps' and the role of ultrasound is to distinguish them apart from testicular neoplasms.

Chapter 8

Thyroid

CASE 1

A 50-year-old woman presents with a painless goitre and is clinically hypothyroid.

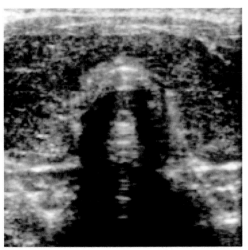

TS thyroid

Q1. What is the diagnosis?

A1. Hashimoto's thyroiditis

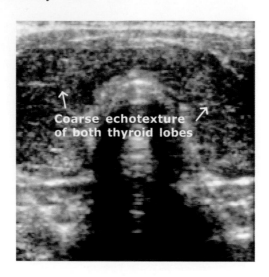

Notes

Hashimoto's thyroiditis is an autoimmune disease which predominantly affects females. In the early stages of the disease patients may be transiently thyrotoxic (hashitoxicosis), but then progress to a hypothyroid state. Clinically they present with a painless firm 'rubbery' goitre.

Ultrasound Features
- Diffusely enlarged gland
- Coarse echo-poor texture (oedema) +/− echo-poor micronodules
- Strong blood flow with colour/power Doppler

Hints

Distinguish from post-viral subacute thyroiditis in which the thyroid gland also appears diffusely echo-poor:

Subacute thyroiditis

Clinical assessment − history of a preceding viral illness, painful tender gland, fever, hyperthyroid state

Ultrasound assessment − absence of colour flow

CASE 2

A 30-year-old woman presents with a swollen neck, palpitations and weight loss. Clinically she has a fine tremor and mild proptosis.

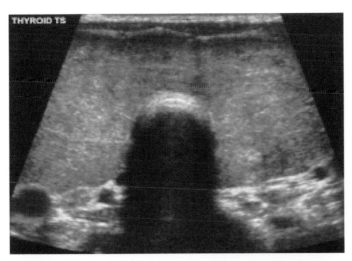

TS thyroid

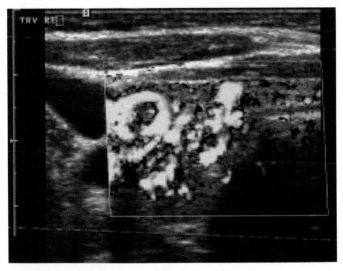

TS right lobe thyroid with power Doppler

Q1. What is the diagnosis?

A1. Graves disease

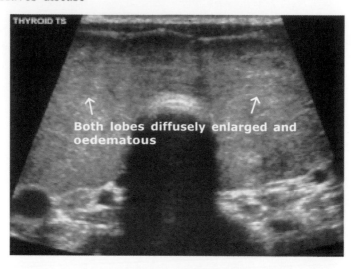

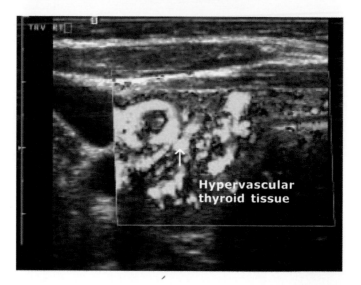

Notes

Graves disease is the commonest cause of hyperthyroidism and is caused by long acting thyroid antibodies which stimulate the gland to release thyroxine. It predominantly affects females and clinically patients have a smooth painless goitre.

Ultrasound Features
- Diffusely enlarged gland
- Normal or echo-poor parenchyma
- Diffusely hypervascular 'thyroid inferno'

Hints
Using spectral Doppler, the peak systolic velocity in the intra-thyroid blood vessels can be measured. Values >50 cm/sec (normal <30 cm/sec) are very suggestive of Graves disease. Normalisation of flow velocities is seen following successful treatment.

CASE 3

A 34-year-old man presents with a firm lump in the right side of his neck. He has a past history of neck irradiation for Hodgkin's disease.

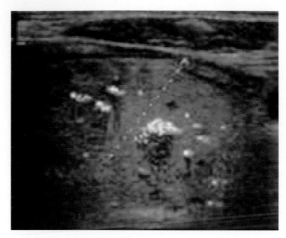

LS right lobe thyroid

Q1. What is the diagnosis?

A1. Thyroid carcinoma (papillary)

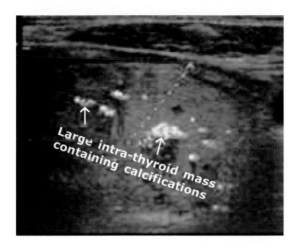

Notes

Head and neck irradiation is the major risk factor for developing thyroid cancer.

Papillary carcinoma is the commonest type, usually affects young adults and spreads early via lymphatics to adjacent neck nodes. It is however a low-grade malignancy and generally has a favourable prognosis. The presence of microcalcifications strongly suggests papillary carcinoma. Other more aggressive thyroid cancers which tend to occur in older patients are follicular carcinoma, lymphoma and anaplastic carcinoma. Medullary thyroid carcinoma is rare and seen in association with multiple endocrine neoplasia (MEN) syndrome type 2.

Ultrasound Features
• Irregular echo-poor mass
• Microcalcifications within the mass (papillary carcinoma)
• Intra-lesional blood flow
• Invasion into surrounding structures, e.g., strap muscles
• Local nodal enlargement

Hints

Image laterally around the carotids and jugular vessels to look for nodal disease.

Any signs suggestive of malignancy warrant a fine needle aspiration (FNA).

Combined ultrasound and FNA are >90% accurate for detecting malignancy.

Cytology cannot distinguish follicular adenoma from carcinoma and surgical removal of the nodule/mass is required.

CASE 4

A 40-year-old man is referred having felt a 'lump' in the right side of his neck.

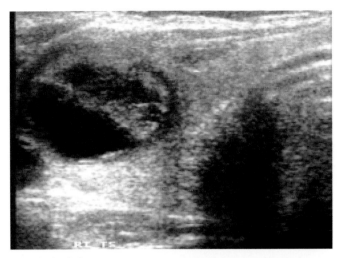

TS right lobe

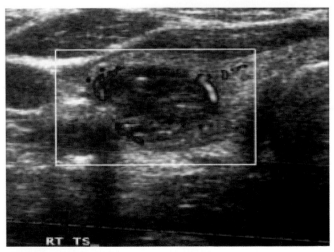

TS right lobe with power Doppler

Q1. What is the diagnosis?
Q2. What is the prognosis?

A1. Solitary thyroid nodule

A2. Likely to be a benign lesion

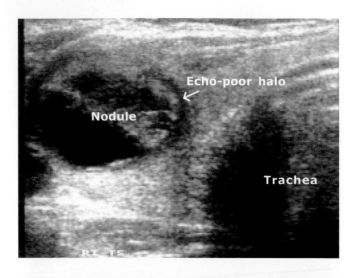

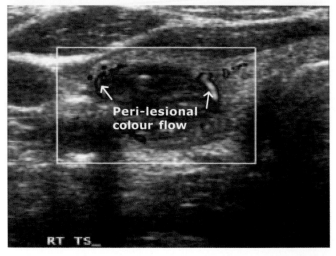

Notes

Thyroid nodules are commonly detected using ultrasound. The majority are benign, but each one requires a thorough assessment. Ultrasound guided needle aspiration can be used to sample suspicious lesions. Solitary adenomas are usually asymptomatic, but occasionally secrete thyroxine causing hyperthyroidism (Plummer's disease).

Ultrasound Features (suggesting a benign nodule)
- Well-defined lesion with a thin echo-poor halo
- Cystic lesion containing 'comet tail' artefacts (colloid)
- Peripheral coarse calcifications
- Peri-lesional blood flow

Hints
Generally speaking if a solitary nodule has no features to suggest malignancy and no risk factors (head and neck irradiation, family history of MEN) it can be followed up with ultrasound to assess for interval change.

CASE 5

A 45-year-old woman presents with a lumpy swelling in her neck. Clinically she is euthyroid.

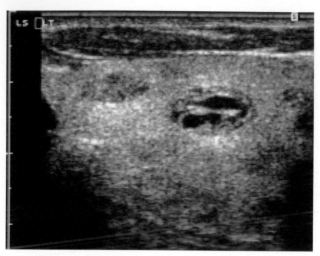

LS left lobe thyroid

Q1. What is the diagnosis?

A1. Multinodular goitre

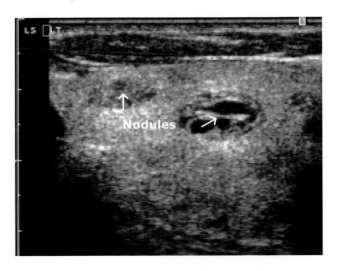

Notes
Multinodular goitre is benign nodular hyperplasia of the thyroid gland which can be hereditary or secondary to iodine deficiency. It is more commonly seen in females and thyroid function tests are usually normal.

Ultrasound Features
- Asymmetrically enlarged gland (AP diameter of a lobe >2 cm).
- Gland contains multiple nodules of different sizes.
- Nodules have a wide variation in appearance: Purely solid, purely cystic or solid/cystic.
- Nodules should not have any malignant features.

Hints
The presence of multiple nodules does not always indicate benign pathology. Thyroid malignancy is commonly multifocal and commonly occurs in association with existent benign nodules. This emphasises the importance of making a thorough assessment of each nodule.

A large goitre with retrosternal extension can cause tracheal compression. To help image the lower pole of each lobe ask the patient to 'blow out their cheeks' which will elevate the gland.

CASE 6

A 35-year-old woman is being investigated for renal stones.

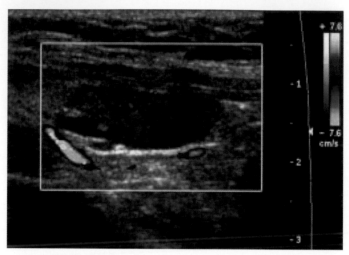

LS left lobe thyroid (lower pole) with colour Doppler

Q1. What is the diagnosis?
Q2. What is the mechanism?

A1. Parathyroid adenoma
A2. Secretion of PTH causing primary hyperparathyroidism

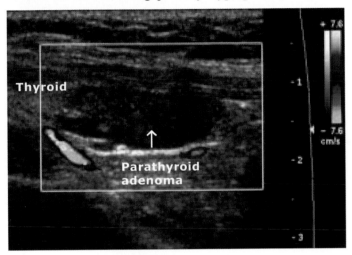

Notes
Parathyroid adenoma is a benign tumour which secretes parathormone (PTH) and is the commonest cause of primary hyperparathyroidism. The resultant hypercalcaemia can cause renal stones, abdominal pain and pancreatitis. Adenomas most commonly arise from the inferior glands.

Ultrasound Features
• Well-defined oblong-shaped echo-poor lesion
• Hypervascular with colour/power Doppler imaging

Hints
There are four parathyroids glands:
Two superior, located posterior to the mid-part of each thyroid lobe.
Two inferior, located posterior to the lower pole of each thyroid lobe.
The normal parathyroid glands are not visible with ultrasound.
10% of parathyroid adenomas may be ectopic within the mediastinum and require scintigraphy or CT/MRI may be required to locate them.

Do not mistake the longus coli muscle or an enlarged neck node for an adenoma.

Secondary hyperparathyroidism (seen in chronic renal failure) typically causes four-gland hyperplasia.

Index